The Pain Didn't Start Here

Susan
Continued Great Mental Wellness

Denyse Hicks-Ray

TSA Communications

The Pain Didn't Start Here

TSA Communications

For further information, contact the author at:

Denyse Hicks-Ray, Ph.D.
P.O. Box 50577
Atlanta, GA 30303-3634
info@traumaservices
www.traumaservices.com
PH: 704-393-3287 or 215-584-1475

Book design by:

The Floating Gallery
244 Madison Ave, #254
New York, NY 10016
877-822-2500
www.thefloatinggallery.com

Printed in Canada

Denyse Hicks-Ray, Ph.D.
The Pain Didn't Start Here

1. Author 2. Title
Library of Congress Control Number: 2004103714
ISBN: 0-9753677-0-6

Acknowledgements

Though I am the sole author of this book, I did not write it alone. Throughout the process, I have been surrounded by family and friends who have supported me in countless ways, and I am grateful.

Long before I began writing in earnest, I shared my vision of the book with my fellow author Marlene Taylor, she continued to encourage me to write one hour a day until there was an outline. She shared my vision and I am grateful. A special thanks to Clarice McGilberry, in the beginning of the building stages Clarice was there when ever I needed something, a true sistah.

First to my sister Diane, thank you for always reading and correcting my written words. But most important, I will always have the gift of you teaching me to read and write before I entered the first grade. You set the foundation for this journey.

To my mentor Dr. Greg Onorato, for advising me to dig deep and search for the answers. You insisted with unabashed enthusiasm that I was a researcher and a healer whether I wanted to admit it or not.

To Melissa Block, my perfect and incredible editor, for your unwavering support, careful shielding, and keen sensibility. There's nothing quite like being on the same page. My gratitude to Larry and Joel my gracious and intelligent publishers, for making it all seem effortless. Your patience with a willful first-time writer has never gone un-noticed.

There were a few that I grew up with, Iman Khairi Shakur, your generous sharing of time and energy showed me this was possible. Kitty Dixon, Talbot's is still my best friend thanks for the introduction.

Rashaan you have always been and continue to be my soul's source of inspiration, ever since that New Years Eve 1974. For you I create a legacy of love, courage and fearlessness. Many hugs and kisses to Qamar and Qailah.

To my best friend and heart Michael, for the greatest book cover design, website, and personal training and most of all your love. Your unfathomable excellence pervades everywhere.

Betty and Joe, I'm so glad we found each other and you joined the journey.

For the Believers:

Commadore & Mother, Albert & Gardenia Tanskley, Freddy & Cynthia Cohen, Rennie, Maurice, Lea, Sonya, Tinita, Heather, Staci, Almitria, D.A Johnson, Mrs. Jarvis, The Staff at Fox Chase Cancer Center, all of my clients and the many people that I have trained. I know you are pleased but not surprised by what I accomplished. To anyone or anything that is not mentioned here, it's only because I have been blessed by so many that my memory is not as great as the gift.

Clearly I have many people to thank, but in addition, I have been continually sustained by the still, small voice I hear when I listen, when I listen carefully. Not by might, not by power, but by spirit alone was I able to finish this book in the time available to me. I felt continually blessed as I wrote it. I hope it is a blessing to those who read it.

"A percent of the proceeds from the book sales will benefit Trauma research and Awareness Campaings throughout the African American community."

Dedicated to the memory of my father, Louis Hicks 1927-2003
Dad, everything good I have inside me you gave me

Table of Contents

Introduction

We, the unwilling, led by the unqualified, have been doing the unbelievable for so long with so little, we now attempt the impossible with nothing.

—Anonymous

If you've picked this book up and opened it, you may consider yourself a trauma survivor. Lord knows there are hundreds of thousands of you out there. If you're like many trauma survivors I've encountered, you're actively searching for answers, seeking solace, seeking help, finding ways to get over whatever was done to you or whatever you witnessed, doing your best to get on with your life. This might be the first book you've looked at on the subject, or it might be the hundredth.

I hope that this book gives you the help you need. This book, however, is not only for you. It is also for the people around you: your family, friends, and community.

Even if you've been fortunate enough to move through life thus far without major trauma, you probably have someone in your life who has been violated in a serious way. Trauma has affected people within your community. Modern communities tend to be fractured and temporary, and when someone within it turns up traumatized, the support network that person needs is often absent. In some instances, people won't acknowledge a traumatized person because they are afraid that they'll say the wrong thing. The trauma survivor feels not only a lack of support, but outright rejection. Fearing this kind of response, many trauma survivors struggle in secret, unwilling to share what they've experienced with others in their community.

Trauma survivors often are treated as malingerers who need to "get over it" and quit feeling sorry for themselves. This attitude, too, silences many a person who desperately needs help and support. Many traumatized people avoid taking the necessary steps to heal themselves because they believe that if they push their pain away for long enough, it will disappear on its own. Or they grow so accustomed to being in pain that they forget how to live without it. That pain becomes a constant companion—an unpleasant one, but at least one that never abandons those who embrace it.

The trauma survivor needs to process and integrate a life-shattering event within a caring and sensitive community. This book will teach you not only how to heal yourself from trauma, but how to be a member of this kind of supportive community.

You may be a therapist or clergyperson who wishes to gain the skills necessary to help traumatized people to move into a healthier space. You may feel lost for words when faced with a child abuser, a murderer, a drug addict, a wife-beater, knowing that you need to feel some kind of compassion in order to help those people, knowing that their pain caused them to do what they have done, knowing that their pain was more likely than not inflicted by similar abuses.

You may be an African-American who wants to understand why people of your race have seemed to fall so far behind in the world in so many ways. You may want to lend support to others like you.

Or, you might be a teacher or a policymaker who seeks to even the playing field in the classroom or in the boardroom, or in the culture at large.

Whoever you are at this moment, I extend to you an invitation to take part in the process of healing African-American pain. This pain has been buried, denied, and ignored for too long. We can no longer bury, deny, or ignore the pain that continues to break the African-American community apart and prevent it from fully participating in the American dream.

Acknowledging this pain will help to heal all of us, because the suffering of any segment of society gives rise to anger and violence. That anger and violence pose a serious threat to those who are in pain, but also to the rest of humanity.

***

In 1996, an internship for my Ph.D. in forensic psychology brought me to a Connecticut prison. I found myself sitting with a woman whose pain I will never forget. At first glance, Danielle (not her real name) didn't seem all that different from me: she was African-American, small and poised, obviously intelligent. There were two very important differences that had put us on opposite sides of the walls of that prison: first, the fact that at only 22 years of age, Danielle had already been convicted of bank robbery; and second, that she had been raped, beaten, and sodomized by her step-father almost daily from the sixth year of her life through the 16th.

Initially, she had an easy time talking with me. When I was able to get her to talk about the abuse she had suffered, however, she became so constricted and frightened by her own pain that she shut down. I wanted to help her heal, so I went to the medical library at the university to see what I could find about therapy for people like Danielle.

When I began to look closely at the literature on psychological trauma, I saw that the modern research and therapeutic guidelines on trauma, post-traumatic stress disorder (PTSD), and its treatment were sorely lacking. I also saw that an understanding of the effects of psychological trauma and a comprehensive approach to treating it is the only way to transform the problem of violence in the African-American community.

I ended up talking with every woman in that Connecticut prison, most of whom were black (as is the case in most U.S. prisons). *Every single woman* incarcerated there presented with signs and symptoms of PTSD. My research at other prisons has revealed the same problem. There isn't a doubt in my mind that a strong link exists between past traumas and present bad behavior.

Since African-Americans make up such a large proportion of people in American prisons, and since they are also more likely to be socioeconomically disadvantaged, this book focuses on the effects of trauma on the issues that are an undeniable part of being African-American. Is our inability to address trauma in the African-American community the reason why such a large portion of it still struggles against enormous obstacles? All the evidence I've seen says yes.

***

Why a book on trauma in the African-American community? I am an African-American myself, one of very few brown faces at the meetings, lectures, and workshops I attend and lead. With such a disproportionate amount of violence being done by and to people of my own race, often upon one another, I feel compelled to address the specific issues that have created this problem. Not many thinkers or therapists have taken this on, and the lack of research into African-American trauma in particular has further alienated an already alienated group of people. Those who need help the most are least able to get it. I see the need for culturally relevant solutions—not solutions designed to erase people's blackness, but solutions that take race and history carefully into account. Current approaches aren't sensitive to African-American culture, and they are woefully inadequate.

No discussion of African-American trauma could be considered complete unless it addresses the role of slavery. When I bring up this point in a room full of white faces, I can see their expressions change from receptive to dubious, so let me explain: I don't bring up the idea that slavery continues to harm modern African-Americans in order to make arguments for reparations or to excuse any of the behaviors that are preventing us from moving forward as a people. I bring it up because cultural trauma is as real as individual trauma, and because we can't deal with individual trauma without addressing the bigger picture.

Historical traumas perpetuate themselves through generations. The factors that create violent children are, more often than not, the factors that create violent adults. These adults go into the world and have more children, and the pain they've packed down from their own childhoods causes them to do the same damage to their children, their lovers, their communities. Slavery, like the Holocaust, is not that far behind us—only one or two or three generations—and to presume that these atrocities don't affect those who are descended from their victims (or from those who were at risk of being victimized because of their race) is just plain wrong.

The men who piloted the planes that killed thousands of people on 9/11 were prime examples of the effects of intergenerational trauma: they were brought up to believe, based on an ages-old territorial conflict, that Zionism is the enemy of good and should be destroyed without mercy. No matter how many terrorists are uprooted, imprisoned, or killed in the so-called War on Terror, more will spring from their ashes, because their children are being taught that they must continue to fight a war against oppression that began centuries ago. They are being taught to hate and to act upon that hate because of perceived injustices that began long before they were born. The only thing that will stop that cycle of violence is understanding where it originated, how it perpetuates itself, and addressing the trauma that has been passed down through the generations.

The same thing needs to be done with African-American youth. Nothing else will stop the gang violence, the shootings, the underachievement, the poverty, the anger that continue to hold us back as a culture and as a race.

In criminal trials, lawyers defend violent criminals by reaching back into their childhoods to prove that they are simply doing unto others as had been done unto them. While this tactic is taken advantage of by some—used to excuse morally repugnant behavior, to remove blame from where it should rightfully be placed—it should not be left out of any discussion of the problem of violence in the African-American community. Any workable solution will consider how today's issues of violence began generations before today's violent criminals were born.

This does not remove blame from such criminals, any more than the centuries of turmoil that motivated the terrorists responsible for 9/11 removed blame from their heads. It does, however, facilitate understanding, and helps us to move towards solutions rather than anger and hatred.

My belief is that psychological trauma in the African-American community is not an issue only for therapists or for those who make laws and make and enforce public policy. It is an issue for anyone who wants to help facilitate a movement away from violence and towards a peaceful, cohesive world where children are safe from harm. My hope is that an understanding of the role trauma plays in the cycle of violence will raise awareness and promote sensitivity in anyone who reads this book.

Since I sat with Danielle in that Connecticut prison, I have stood witness as trauma survivors have devised incredible ways to protect themselves and relieve some of the pain they have endured. This movement towards safety, this struggle for inner peace, carries with it its own unique energy. When one sits with a survivor and feels the strength involved in simply going on, it's difficult not to feel awe and respect for their struggle. I have felt so inspired by the strength and dignity I see in these people that I became committed to helping trauma sufferers—in the words of William Faulkner—"not to endure, but to prevail."

Our deepest fear is not that we are inadequate. Our deepest fear is that we are powerful beyond measure. It's our light, not our darkness that most frightens us. We ask ourselves, who am I to be brilliant, gorgeous, talented, and fabulous?

—Nelson Mandela

Chapter One

Trauma: What It Is, What It Isn't

Every day's news brings new reports of violence done by children:

- In New Jersey, an 11-year-old boy was sentenced to 18 years in the custody of the juvenile justice system for fatally beating a three-year-old with a baseball bat and dumping him face-down in a drainage ditch. The boy told the judge that he had done this because the toddler was bothering him and wanted to use his scooter.
- A gang member fatally shot two high school students while trying to kill a rival gang member, who he spotted running up a staircase some distance away.
- In Fall of 2003, a 15-year-old boy shot a student athlete to death. In court, he described the shooting as unintentional, because he had meant to shoot at two other people who were present.
- In September of 1997, a 16-year-old New Jersey boy raped and strangled an 11-year-old boy to death.
- According to US Department of Justice statistics, 16 percent of forcible rape arrestees in 1997 were juveniles. Seventeen percent of those arrested for other sex offenses that year were juveniles as well.
- A ten-year-old boy employed his three-year-old niece as a shield against a sheriff's deputy, at whom he was aiming a gun.

- A high school soccer star was forced to transfer to another school because of bullying and death threats from his classmates.
- At one Manhattan primary school, a group of children wearing ski masks charged into a classroom and stole a student's jacket and money, beating him up in the process. At the same school, safety agents were attacked by three students, and a vending machine was thrown down a flight of stairs.

Heads shake, tongues cluck, heavy sighs are breathed. "What's *wrong* with children nowadays?" we ask. "What could cause a child to do this kind of harm to others?" Children are supposed to be good, they are supposed to be pure.

The answers range far and wide: violent rap lyrics, violent video games and movies, overt sexuality in the media, absent parents, incompetent parents, lack of community, the influence of drugs or alcohol, premature sexuality, poor nutrition, socioeconomic inequality, prejudice, racism, lack of motivation to do right instead of wrong, lack of discipline, lack of self-esteem, rampant materialism. When we begin to catalogue the possible explanations for violence in American children, we might begin to wonder why *more* of them don't strike out.

There is no shortage of news on violence in the African-American community, either. Most of it is black-on-black: young black men full of promise struck down by bullets while going about their daily lives, or gang members or bystanders caught up in the drama of gang warfare. African-American men are seven times more likely to die in a homicide than white men. Black women face less risk, but it's still four times that of their white counterparts. It's unbearably sad and totally futile, and again we wonder how this could be happening—and, at the same time, when we truly appreciate the problems of socioeconomic inequality and racial prejudice, we wonder why the problems aren't worse than they are.

Each of the factors that plays a role in creating violent children plays an equally strong role in creating violent adults. No treatise on violence in children would be complete without a close look at the adults they become, the adults who shape them, and, in turn, what made those influential adults into who they are today. One important root cause of violence in children—and in the adults that they become—is childhood trauma.

All of the factors listed at the beginning of this chapter also play roles in increasing rates of depression, anxiety, and self-destructive behaviors in both children and adults. Each needs to be addressed. Each of the contributing factors I listed helps to create an environment where trauma is more likely. Many of those factors make processing of and healing from trauma more difficult.

The idea that trauma in childhood can give rise to psychological illness has passed in and out of vogue a few times since Sigmund Freud first linked childhood sexual abuse with "hysterical" symptoms in women. Most of the women he treated with talk therapy for these unexplainable psychosomatic symptoms turned out to have been abused sexually as children. Contrary to the popular belief that only lower-class, poor people were guilty of taking advantage of young girls in this way, many of the women Freud treated were from the most esteemed, highest-class families in Vienna. Freud knew that any theory that blamed sexual abuse for hysteria would reveal an enormous amount of sexual abuse going on in all levels of society. He knew that the backlash would erase his credibility, and he quickly abandoned that aspect of his research.

Even today, the suggestion that trauma is what causes children to become violent is controversial. The suggestion that African-American children are traumatized by long-standing socioeconomic inequality and racism between blacks and whites is difficult to refute, but even more difficult to address head-on. The problems begin to seem so vast, the solutions so unattainable. But look we must, because acknowledgement is remarkably healing in and of itself. Acknowledgement of trauma and its pervasive effects is an indispensable part of the healing process, the one that has to happen before the rest of the process is possible.

It is hard to take a clear look at the serious divisions—divisions of color, wealth, status, and power—that continue to plague our privileged nation and plant the seeds of violence. It is hard to look at the evils so-called "civilized" people continue to perpetrate on one another. No one wants to take the blame for creating divisions or doing harm, but a great many people are looking for somewhere to heap that blame.

If we wish to help those who have survived traumatic events, we must be willing to face and acknowledge what we feel to be unspeakable. We need to understand what exactly constitutes a traumatic event, and how such an event changes the person who goes through it. We need to share the burden of terror and anguish carried by those who have been traumatized. Only then can we learn to support trauma survivors the way they need to be supported in order to heal. Only then can those who have suffered traumatic events become part of the solution instead of the problem.

This understanding also allows us to see how trauma has affected us personally, and how to move out of whatever damage that trauma has done.

Working Definition of Trauma

What it all comes down to is pain.

Pain so deep that it causes you to not treat your children right, to be unable to be in a healthy love relationship,. Pain that causes you to think ill of others when you have yet to take a look at your own errors. This is ; the kind of pain that comes from a violation of the order of your universe, from a trauma intense enough to make you question the foundations of your beliefs. I have heard hundreds of people say, "I can't believe that this could happen to me," but these words have never lost their poignancy. What they really mean is: *My world no longer makes sense.*

How often have you heard someone say that he's been "traumatized" by an event? This expression has entered the pop culture mainstream, but let's talk about what it really means. *The essence of trauma is the loss of faith that there is order and continuity in life.* Following a traumatic experience, we see that the world is not what we thought it was, that the foundations upon which we have built our view of self and others are crumbled or crumbling. Any painful or frightening emotional or physical experience, including parental abandonment, parental abuse, sexual assault, war, or natural disasters, can be considered traumatic.

A traumatic event involves actual or threatened injury or death to self or others. Overwhelming force robs the trauma victim of control and power. Her emotional reaction to the event overtakes her ability to cope in that moment. It instills intense fear, helplessness, and horror, and undermines the sense of security that comes from knowing what to expect from one's world. For months, years, or even decades following the experience, many trauma survivors suffer the repercussions of that overwhelming moment.

Trauma need not be a life-threatening event; it can be the result of betrayal by trusted or needed people or institutions. The events of September 11th, 2001 traumatized the entire U.S. and people all over the world. It's hard to imagine a person who has not at least been touched by severe trauma in his or her lifetime.

For example:

A child witnesses a gang shooting.

A family is almost decimated by a house fire.

A pregnant woman has a difficult labor and emergency Caesarian section.

A nation watches, over and over again, news footage of doomed people leaping from the top floors of the burning World Trade Towers on 9/11.

A child watches as her close relative dies of cancer.

A woman survives internment in a concentration camp.

A young man commits murder; both he and those who witnessed the murder are traumatized.

A previously healthy person develops a painful chronic intestinal disorder.

A soldier overseas witnesses the deaths of several of his comrades before being shot by an enemy soldier.

A child is sexually abused by a relative or family friend, once or repeatedly.

A child is abandoned by his father or mother.

A mother loses a child to gang violence.

An infant is left to cry as its parents smoke heroin in the next room.

Trauma can consist of a single event or repeated events. Some traumas, such as chronic illness, come and go for years or even a lifetime, re-traumatizing the individual again and again. A traumatic event in childhood predisposes the survivor to re-traumatization later in life. Dr. Judith Herman, a psychiatrist and author of the classic work *Trauma and Recovery,* points out that "traumatic events are extraordinary, not because they occur rarely, but rather because they overwhelm the ordinary human adaptations to life."

The common denominator of all traumatic events is the fallout that affects nearly all those who experience them. This fallout varies dramatically from person to person.

Some people seem wired to handle trauma better than others. I've seen people who were traumatized by events that others could overcome without difficulty. This is not necessarily dependent on that person's strength or weakness (in fact, the "stronger" the person, the more likely they'll be to avoid dealing with traumatic events and to end up with post-traumatic stress), but more on their emotional and psychological makeup.

According to Carl Bell, M.D., an African-American physician and a leading theorist on trauma's effects on children, the key factor is something called *resiliency.* A resilient person has inner resources and attitudes that enable him to endure extreme circumstances and to bounce back afterwards without lasting damage. Resiliency will be discussed in greater detail in chapters to come.

Those who choose occupations that repeatedly expose them to trauma—doctors, firefighters, policemen, EMTs, soldiers—tend to be people who are better able to handle life-and-death situations. They develop ways of compartmentalizing and dealing with what they see from day to day, and this does lead to post-traumatic stress syndrome in some of them. One important avenue of trauma research is to help prevent PTSD in those who are there for us in our moments of danger.

During the Traumatic Event

What happens to the brain and body during trauma that has such devastating effects in its aftermath? Danger of any kind evokes an ages-old, deeply ingrained response that involves both the nervous and endocrine (hormonal) systems. Pupils dilate, heart rate and blood pressure increase, sense organs reach their peak of sensitivity, reaction time shortens, and attention narrows to the situation at hand. Fear and anger are typical emotional responses to danger. These physical and emotional reactions allow us to overcome hunger, pain, or fatigue, and enable us to protect ourselves from danger by fighting or fleeing. Collectively, they are known as the *stress response.*

Helplessness and loss of control distinguish simple stress from trauma. In traumatic situations, the stress response kicks in just as it should, but it has no impact on the event that is occurring. No matter how hard the victim tries to fight or flee, there is no escape. Again, to quote Dr. Herman: "When neither resistance nor escape is possible, the human system of self-defense becomes overwhelmed and disorganized. Each component…tends to persist in an altered and exaggerated state long after the actual danger is over."

The memories formed during trauma are unlike those formed during happier moments, or even during times of stress. Adrenaline and other "fight-or-flight" hormones are at their highest levels when we are most threatened, and helplessness prevents us from acting upon the urges they bring out in us. This potent mix of biochemicals changes the way we remember. In the moment of traumatic experience, the person may dissociate, effectively separating herself from an unbearable experience that she can escape in no other way. Sensations of pain and fear dissipate and the trauma victim may see the rest of the event from outside of himself. Sexually abused children have been known to "put themselves in the wall" during episodes of abuse, and rape victims often report having watched the event from outside of their own bodies—removing themselves so that they don't have to suffer quite so much.

Dissociation is protective in those moments of incomprehensible fear and helplessness. However, the long-term effects of dissociation can be serious if the trauma survivor does not seek to reunite his memories with his consciousness. The intensity of the dissociation response is a strong predictor of whether the trauma survivor will have post-traumatic stress.

Creation of memories is strongly affected by dissociation. Traumatic memories are stored as vivid imagery, fragments of sensory information and emotion. They come up in the form of dissociated images and sensations. A survivor of sexual abuse might only remember the appearance of the face of her abuser during their encounters; a soldier might only recall the smell of decaying corpses on the battlefield; a survivor of a flood might only feel terror whenever he has to go near a body of water. These trauma survivors may not recall the actual event at all, or only vaguely; there may only be terrifying flashes and hints of the experience that caused them to dissociate.

Post-Traumatic Stress Disorder

Most of the people I have treated for post-traumatic stress tell me at some point that they are ashamed of their weakness, their inability to overcome the traumatic event. They feel that there is something fundamentally wrong with them. I tell these patients that they are *reacting normally to an abnormal situation.* Once the survivor stops blaming himself, the healing can begin.

On the flip side of the coin, there are trauma survivors who focus intently on blaming others for their misfortunes. Young men in prison often tell me, "I had to kill him before he killed me." I've heard all kinds of bad behavior blamed on all kinds of people, but the bottom line is that blaming stands in the way of healing from trauma, too—especially when the blame is placed on some person or circumstance that really has nothing to do with the real, underlying issue: the fact that this young man was beaten every day by his father during his childhood, or that he witnessed a shooting, or that his mother was a drug addict who left him to fend for himself before he was able to do without her.

The so-called "symptoms" that often follow a traumatic event are *not* abnormal. They are adaptations designed by Nature to protect the trauma survivor from further exposure to dangerous situations—adaptations that allow that person to cope when her usual coping mechanisms are overwhelmed. After all, a mother who has survived a rape has to go on mothering her children; the soldier back from war has to hold a job and support his family; the teenager who has been assaulted must go to school and be with peers; the child who has been sexually abused by her stepfather must go on living with her parents (or so she believes, feeling that she is safer there than in another home away from her abuser). Life does go on.

The problem is that trauma eats away at us until we can no longer manage even the simplest daily responsibilities. It causes us to make a mess of child-rearing and relationships. Until trauma is acknowledged and integrated, it will be perpetuated.

African-Americans are More Vulnerable to Trauma

The problems faced by much of the African-American community create an environment that breeds stress and trauma. More blacks live in poverty and in inner cities. They face prejudice and barriers to socioeconomic equality at every turn. Their history in this country began with slavery, which gave way to decades of segregation and racial prejudice that only since the 1980s have begun to lift. Some would argue that blacks continue to be exploited, subjugated, and treated unequally compared with whites. While whites have had the means to accumulate wealth and power since they first settled this continent, most blacks have been held back from doing so until very recently. No amount of affirmative action or social programming has made up for this handicap.

Black culture has not assimilated. Assimilation describes a gradual replacement of a culture's history, traits, and traditions with those of the mainstream culture. In the face of pressures to dissolve into the mainstream white culture, black culture has retained its strength, its uniqueness, its beauty. African-Americans are caught between the need for assimilation—which, theoretically, allows them to gain the advantages that the majority enjoys—and the desire to hang on to and evolve the gifts of their ancestors. The modern arts of hip-hop and rap have their roots in Africa and other largely black nations. Its mainstreaming into white American culture seems at first like a success on the part of African-American culture, but as we will see later in this book, it's not always as good a thing for black folks as we might want to believe.

Economic inequality breeds violence more than racial differences, as shown by an analysis of 125 major American metropolitan areas by sociologists Judith and Peter Blau. They found that all types of violent crime are strongly associated with levels of inequality between the top and bottom levels of the socioeconomic scale. In other words: those who find themselves poor because of factors out of their control—not education, or income, but skin color—are more prone to anger, hostility, and violence towards others. This violence is usually wrought on people of the same race, which compounds the fear and distrust African-Americans live with every day.

African-Americans are more likely to have disorganized families. By 1990, only 36 percent of black children lived with both parents. African-American men are less able to pull their children out of poverty even when they are in the home with them. They have higher rates of death than whites for the 15 leading causes of death in the U.S., with the exceptions of lung disease and suicide.

Without a doubt, traumatic situations spring more easily from this kind of soil. When security and senses of order and control are already so precarious, it takes little disruption to throw a child off-balance. Those children become traumatized adults. In African-American culture, those who would seek to undergo the long process of acknowledging and healing trauma are less respected than those who appear to overcome it right away and move on.

The more difficult a trauma survivor's everyday circumstances, the more strength she has to muster in order to get on with her life. A single mother who is living in poverty, holding down two jobs just to make ends meet, is going to have to be far more adept at burying the aftereffects of trauma than a woman who lives in a more financially comfortable, relaxed situation. The poorer woman is also going to have a much harder time getting the right kind of professional help, and is far less likely to even believe that such help is necessary or available.

This is one source of the stereotype of the poor, stoic, long-suffering African-American woman who sets her jaw and does what she has to do. Unfortunately, the seeming strength of these women perpetuates resistance against healing trauma and post-traumatic stress in themselves and in their children.

Post-Traumatic Stress Disorder

The natural reactions to traumatic stress become post-traumatic stress disorder (PTSD) when they cause significant distress or impairment. A diagnosis of PTSD is made when the following symptoms are present for at least one month, and when they interfere with the person's ability to live, love and work normally: *intrusions, avoidance, constriction,* and *hyperarousal.*

Intrusions

Intrusions may include flashbacks, nightmares, or other re-experiencing of the trauma. They interfere with everyday life, affecting sleep and causing the trauma survivor to feel as if he can't control his thoughts. His mind continues to flash to the event that caused him so much pain and terror. Intrusions can stifle appropriate development in traumatized children, as they become "frozen" in time at the point of the traumatic event.

Avoidance

The trauma survivor avoids people or things that might bring on intrusive symptoms. Any situation or person that might remind the survivor of her trauma is carefully avoided, either by physically staying away from places or people that bring up intrusive memories or by dissociating. Those who have a tendency to dissociate—to remove themselves from what's happening, to compartmentalize traumatic experience and not integrate it—seem more vulnerable to PTSD. (I will talk in detail about dissociation in Chapter Five.)

Avoidance also prevents trauma survivors from seeking therapy. Therapy seeks to bring all of the issues to the surface that most traumatized people would much rather try to bury.

Constriction

Constriction begins during the trauma itself as the person begins to feel as though he is standing outside of his body, as though he has become detached from the whole situation. He may feel indifferent, sinking into passivity rather than continuing to struggle against unbeatable odds. Sensations are altered and physical pain may not be felt at all.

Trauma survivors often continue to feel helpless after their trauma has ended. Unable to fight or flee, they froze, and the thaw may not be complete for months, years, or decades. They "shut down," altering their own states of consciousness in an effort to protect themselves against further harm. They are able to wall off painful recollections from everyday thoughts and experiences. Trauma survivors may also begin to limit the things they do, the places they go, and the people they communicate with in an effort to feel safe. They may stop thinking about the future.

Intrusions, avoidance, and constriction tend to become enmeshed in a downward spiral that moves the trauma survivor away from love, peace, and fulfillment. She takes on avoidance behaviors to avoid the intrusions, and her world constricts as a result.

Some trauma survivors alternate between avoidance and intentional placing of themselves "at the scene of the crime." For example, women who were sexually abused as children may seek out abusive partners when they reach adulthood. A man who has been assaulted in a bad neighborhood may continue to return to that neighborhood to prove he isn't afraid to do so. Most psychologists agree that these behaviors are unconscious attempts to heal through reliving of the trauma.

Hyperarousal

Hyperarousal, also known as *hypervigilance,* describes the physical condition of a person who is on the edge, expecting danger at every turn—even when there's no reason to be afraid or anxious. A hyperaroused person is tense and startles easily.

During and in the aftermath of World War I, psychologists began to study "shell-shock," where soldiers who were exposed to gruesome or treacherous battle situations became as unhinged as the hysterical women studied by Freud and Breuer. At first, it was believed that shell-shock was caused by the sounds of shells exploding, but later it was recognized as a more complex problem caused by repeated, prolonged exposure to life-threatening violence. Those who have been traumatized by battle situations may always be prepared to do battle again, reacting violently to loud noises or stressful situations.

A child exposed to gang warfare or domestic violence is likely to be hyperaroused. Increased arousal does more than increase tendency to violent behavior; it also decreases a person's ability to pay attention. Children with PTSD are often misdiagnosed with learning disabilities or attention deficit/hyperactivity disorder (ADHD) because they're too fearful to pay attention in school.

Hyperarousal is one of the most important reasons why children become violent. Boys who have been traumatized feel soothed when they commit violent acts against others. Their feelings of power and control are restored by these acts. Girls tend not to do violence against others; they tend more towards self-destructive behaviors and self-mutilation ("cutting"), both of which seem to have the same soothing effects in the aftermath of trauma.

Other Symptoms of Post-Traumatic Stress

As long as the terror, hatred, and rage of the moment of trauma remain unhealed, they bleed into the trauma survivor's life in the form of PTSD symptoms. Other common symptoms that appear following a psychological trauma include depression and anxiety. Treatment of depression and anxiety with medications—without also implementing talk therapy and the other steps outlined in the second half of this book—further remove trauma survivors from facing what they've gone through, integrating it into their selves and their lives, and moving on. Medication to ease anxiety or depression can be helpful in the short-term; We'll talk about that later in Chapter five.

Dissociation and *somatoform disorders,* unexplained physical symptoms that can be linked back to a traumatic event, are also common. A whole spectrum of dissociative disorders has been defined, and you will learn more about this fascinating field in Chapter Five. Victimization is also common, and this will be discussed in more detail in Chapter three [community trauma, post slavery syndrome]. Suicide risk is high in trauma survivors. In one study of women who were raped, nearly one in five attempted suicide in the years following.

PTSD symptoms tend to change over the course of time. Symptoms can arise and disappear, or be transformed into new symptoms as the days, weeks, months, and years pass. It is an unpredictable disorder. As you might imagine, all of these symptoms, individually or combined, disconnects the individual from his community. PTSD robs people of the support they so desperately need by making them unable or unwilling to relate to others. This is a crucial point, reminding us of the role of the community in bringing trauma survivors back from the brink.

Chapter Two

From Freud to Bell and Back Again
A History of the Diagnosis and Treatment of Trauma

"*...History is more than the record of man's conflict with nature and himself. It is the knowledge which gives dimension to the present, direction to the future, and humility to the leaders of men. A nation, like a person, not conscious of its own past is adrift without purpose or protection against the contending forces of dissolution.*"

—Lyndon B. Johnson, spoken on the first anniversary of the death of John F. Kennedy, November 22, 1964

Literature, theater, music, and the visual arts have all been used to chronicle traumatic episodes since the beginnings of history. Think of Medea, who murdered her own children to punish an unfaithful husband. Hamlet's crisis and murders come in response to the untimely murder of his father by his ambitious uncle. Romeo and Juliet both die because of the war between their families, which has gone on for generations.

Where there is trauma, there is drama, and the media of today—films, television, popular music—work on this same premise. The modern movie that doesn't involve some kind of trauma is rare indeed.

Artists have long recognized the value of capturing moments of horror on canvas, on film, or in whatever other media they choose: those who view their work are brought into that moment of terror, united with all others who viewed them before. By creating art that reflects traumatic events, artists catalyze the integration of those events into the collective consciousness. Art helps to fulfill the human drive to deal with and move past traumatic events.

Although trauma has been around as long as human beings have walked the earth, and although that trauma has been chronicled in the arts for nearly as long, the scientific study of trauma has been sporadic and controversial. Troublesome issues abound in the study of trauma. Who is to blame and who is the victim? How about those who have seemed to block out a past trauma—usually an episode or episodes of sexual abuse—and who then "recover" memories of that abuse? Can such memories be "planted" by those who do not necessarily have the patient's best interest at heart? Whose responsibility is it to help traumatized people heal and become more productive members of society?

These questions have no easy answers, and healing trauma on a broad level requires that we begin to address them. According to Bessel Van der Kolk, "submitting impulses for revenge to the arbitration of the rule of law, finding common symbols and memorials, establishing agencies responsible for social security, and honoring and identifying with people who are symbols of righteousness—all these issues present particular challenges to societies that have been marked by oppression and brutality." (*Traumatic Stress,* p.40) It's hard to think of any society that has not at some point either brutalized or been brutalized by others.

Hysteria: The Root of Modern Trauma Theory

Jean-Martin Charcot (1825-1893) was the first scientist to define and study a disorder that had been known for centuries as *hysteria.* Hysterical patients presented with one or more of the following symptoms:

Paralysis (usually partial)
Blindness
Deafness
Amnesia

Pain or other body sensations for which no physical cause could be found
Contracture of the limbs (difficulty moving because of tightened muscles)
Mutism (inability to speak)
Limping
Nightmares
Insomnia
Heart palpitations
Dizziness
Depression
Disorientation
"Fits" of fainting
Fearful outbursts

Hysteria is a term derived from the Greek word for uterus. Until the middle of the 20th century, it was believed to be a distinctly female condition, biologically based in some aspect of her reproductive organs. The term eventually became an all-inclusive diagnosis that was not backed by any scientific definition, one that encompassed every so-called "female problem," from frigidity to nymphomania to spinsterism to work done towards women's rights!

By dismissing so many of women's issues, dreams, and desires as the result of a pathological condition—one that arose from their biological makeup, their "weak constitutions"— men were able to continue to subjugate their wives, sisters, daughters, and mothers until the women's liberation movement gained real momentum in the 1970s.

Hysteria was first described in ancient Egypt, around 1900 B.C. Hysterical symptoms were ascribed to "displacement of the uterus." If the uterus floated too high in the body, it was thought to affect the brain. Hippocrates recommended that hysterical women inhale noxious odors, which he theorized would push the organ back down to its proper location. Bloodletting was also used to treat hysterical symptoms in those days.

Hippocrates also believed that hysteria was caused by sexual deprivation, a notion that lasted well into the 20th century in more liberal-minded circles. In fact, genital massage was once a popular treatment for mental illness in women. The earliest vibrators were created to relieve physicians of the arduous task of massaging female patients to "hysterical paroxysm," which seemed to help relieve all sorts of symptoms.

In the Middle Ages, hysterical symptoms were attributed to demonic possession, witchcraft, or religious fanaticism. Up until the 19th century, women were subjected to exorcism and witch hunts throughout the world. Some tried to treat hysteria more gently, with strength-building diets and bed rest, but as soon as surgery became a viable option, a good number of unnecessary ophorectomies (removal of the ovaries) and hysterectomies (removal of the uterus) were performed in an effort to cure hysterical women.

Other early therapeutic recommendations included beatings with a wet towel, suffocation (until a hysterical "fit" was calmed), and electroshock. It was believed by some that hysterical women were faking their symptoms in an effort to get attention. Chastisement and shaming were the therapies of choice in these situations. Even after Charcot's work had become well-known, none of the cures that had been tried were considered to have been successful.

Charcot worked at the Salpêtriére, a women's mental hospital in Paris, France. He treated women who were poor and had often been subjected to plenty of abuse, both sexual and non-sexual. In his famous "Tuesday lectures," he would perform dramatic demonstrations, placing subjects under hypnosis and displaying their hysterical symptoms to rapt audiences that included doctors and wealthy laypeople. In the end, Charcot concluded that hysteria was a degenerative "functional disease of the nervous system" that was caused by a combination of constitution and heredity. He did not believe that there was a cure.

One of Charcot's students, Sigmund Freud, would find out—along with colleague Josef Breuer and another scientist named Pierre Janet—why Charcot hadn't been able to cure his patients: he treated them as subjects to place under a microscope, but he didn't think to *talk* to them, or to try to get them to talk to him.

The Talking Cure: Freud, Breuer, and Janet

Pierre Janet was Charcot's successor at the Salpêtriére. Janet began to see that the weakened constitution that seemed to make way for the onset of hysterical symptoms had something to do with trauma:

I was led to recognize in certain cases the role of one or several events in the subject's past life. These events, which had established a violent emotion and a destruction of the psychological system, had left traces. The remembrance of these events, the mental work involved in their recall and settlement, persisted in the form of lower and more or less conscious psychological processes, absorbed a great deal of strength, and played a part in the persistent weakening.

—from Murchison, Carl, *History of Psychology in Autobiography,* Vol. 1, Clark University Press, Worcester, MA, 1930: p.123-133.

In 1885, ten years before Charcot's death, Sigmund Freud was a struggling research scientist who could barely make ends meet. Some of his less remarkable early work included a treatise on the benefits of cocaine. (He was one of many scientists who recommended this drug for all kinds of ailments.) A six-month stay in Paris at the Salpêtriére inspired him to wholeheartedly embrace the study of psychopathology, the science of mental illness. Freud's colleague, Josef Breuer, joined him in working with hypnosis to find the causes of—and cure for—hysteria.

One of Breuer's patients, known to the world then as Anna O, was probably the most famous hysteric in history. At 21, she collapsed one day while nursing her dying father. She then developed a squint and a nervous cough, and sometimes seemed unable to speak. She would have hallucinations of her fingers turning into snakes or of snakes attacking her father, but only during the day; at night, she spontaneously fell into a trance. Her right arm and neck would become paralyzed. She would reply to questions in French, English, or Italian instead of her native German. Anna O. also developed an alternate personality that was exactly one year younger than her "real" personality.

Breuer was able to hypnotize Anna O. During their sessions, Breuer found that when he could get his patient to reveal the cause of a symptom, the symptom would disappear. For example, she told him that when her dying father had asked her the time, she had not been able to see the face of the watch through her tears, and had to squint. Once she had told this story to Breuer, her squint disappeared. Breuer called this the *cathartic method,* but Anna called it "the talking cure." Together with Freud, Breuer authored *Studies on Hysteria,* which outlined the cathartic method. It was published in 1896, and was the first work to try to establish hysteria not as a physiological condition, but as a psychological one.

Anna and Breuer met every day for more than a year. The patient, understandably, grew very dependent upon the doctor, and her symptoms got worse if he could not see her, even if his substitute used the same techniques. After a while, it became obvious that Anna had fallen in love with Breuer, and even believed herself to be pregnant with his child. She was not pregnant at all, and Breuer was a married man; still, his realization that he had grown quite attached to her as well drove him to stop meeting with her altogether. Anna was not cured at that point, and spent a few more years in mental hospitals before going out into the world and becoming a highly respected feminist activist. She revealed her true name, Bertha Pappenheim, and spent the rest of her life fighting for the rights of women and Jews around the world.

Meanwhile, Freud was doing similar work with his own patients. He found that letting his patients talk freely revealed just as much as hypnosis. Nearly every one of Freud's patients had recollections of a sexual experience during childhood, and they were all reluctant to talk about that experience. When persuaded to tell Freud about it, they became upset, but once they had finished telling the story, they felt relief. Freud concluded that early sexual experience was the common denominator linking hysterical women.

According to Freud, symptoms rarely showed up during childhood. He claimed that this was due to the suppression of the memory of the sexual experience, along with the intense emotions that accompanied the experience. (Today we know that sexually abused children are just as likely to manifest signs of post-traumatic stress as adults—they just manifest them differently.) During talk therapy, these women resisted the resurfacing of the memories and emotions that were at the root of their hysterical symptoms. Freud saw that in order to treat hysterical women, he would need to breach that resistance and persuade them to reveal what had happened to them.

In Freud's own words, spoken at a lecture that was published in the *American Journal of Psychiatry:*

"Suppose that here in this hall and in this audience, whose exemplary stillness and attention I cannot sufficiently commend, there is an individual who is creating a disturbance, and, by his ill-bred laughing, talking, by scraping his feet, distracts my attention from my task. I explain that I cannot go on with my lecture under these conditions, and thereupon several strong men among you get up, and, after a short struggle, eject the disturber of the peace from the hall. He is now 'repressed,' and I can continue my lecture. But in order that the disturbance may not be repeated, in case the man who has just been thrown out attempts to force his way back into the room, the gentlemen who have executed my suggestion take their chairs to the door and establish themselves as a 'resistance,' to keep up the repression. Now, if you transfer both locations to the psyche, calling this 'consciousness,' and the outside the 'unconscious,' you have a tolerably good illustration of the process of repression...

"Remember that with the ejection of the rowdy and the establishment of the watchers before the door, the affair is not necessarily ended. It may very well happen that the ejected man, now embittered and quite careless of consequences, gives us more to do. He is no longer among us, we are free from his presence, his scornful laugh, his half-audible remarks, but in a certain sense the repression has miscarried, for he makes a terrible uproar outside, and by his outcries and by hammering on the door with his fists interferes with my lecture more than before."

—Sigmund Freud, "The Origin and Development of Psychoanalysis," *American Journal of Psychiatry,* 21:181-218.

Freud's work was the beginning of modern trauma theory, but Freud's theories about the conscious and subconscious minds did not originate with him. It had long been believed that a part of the mind was inaccessible to workaday thought but was delved into during dreams and altered states of consciousness. In the years before Freud became famous, a psychologist named Fechner described the unconscious (also known as the subconscious) mind as an iceberg—more specifically, as the enormous, hidden part beneath the surface. Repressed memories were pushed into the unconscious, but the power of those memories would bleed into the conscious mind.

If sexual abuse had been behind every case of hysteria, and if medicine and the general public were expected to accept this, it would have to be accepted that the sexual abuse of children was practically epidemic within every level of society. Freud saw that this would never fly, and so he repudiated that aspect of his theory—one that had been a major part of *The Aetiology of Hysteria*—and began to explore the "frustrated desires" of hysterics. He began to claim that the women who reported childhood sexual abuse were actually making their stories up.

According to this line of reasoning, his patients were disturbed by their own unfulfilled sexual urges and fantasies, not by traumatic rapes or molestations during their formative years. From that point forward, Freud ceased to be a champion for women and entered the hallowed halls of misogyny. His became the dominant psychological theory for nearly a century. The damage this did to the ability of women to seek effective help for healing from traumatic events lasted for nearly as long.

Shell-Shock and the Trauma of War

In World War I, ten million young men died in battle and 20 million others died of hunger and disease brought about by the war. [Howard Zinn, *A People's History of the United States: 1492-present,* HarperCollins Perennial Classics, New York, NY 1999.] The amount of killing that went on in WWI is still hard to comprehend; within the first months of the war, almost every man who had come to fight in the original ranks of the British army was dead.

Americans were sent into the fray in 1917, three years after the war began. Young Americans weren't exactly eager to take part in this "war to end all wars," and so the government instituted a draft and a propaganda campaign designed to persuade the nation that its involvement in this bloody war was a good and right thing. By November 1918, the war had ended and 50,000 American soldiers had died.

Those who survived the war were left haunted by the memory of what they had seen, heard, smelled, and felt during their service.

During the war itself, men began to break down, behaving like hysterical women: crying uncontrollably, or losing their ability to move or speak, or falling apart in other ways that made them useless to their comrades at the front. This was especially common in soldiers who spent days or weeks at a time fighting in the trenches.

At first, shell-shocked soldiers were thought to have been damaged by the sounds of shells exploding. It soon became obvious that this wasn't the problem, because men who had not been anywhere near exploding shells were presenting with the same symptoms as those who had. The official name of the collection of symptoms then became *combat neurosis,* but the original term is still used to describe extreme reactions to traumatic events.

Early theories about treating combat neurosis revolved around the idea that men who succumbed to it were somehow morally inferior. It was believed that these men needed to be berated and threatened until they snapped out of it, after which point they could go right back to fight with their units. British therapist Lewis Yealland made a name for himself by brow-beating shell-shocked soldiers. In addition to shaming and threats of court-martial, electric shocks and repetition of patriotic slogans were used to try to prop up these devastated men long enough to go and face the same horrors again.

Fortunately, more humane treatments were suggested by a group of therapists that included Abram Kardiner, an American schooled on psychoanalytic principles in Vienna. Kardiner's research and treatments were the beginnings of the modern methods used to treat those who have undergone life-shattering traumas.

In every war, both soldiers and civilians are traumatized. World War II and Korea were not exceptions, but interest in helping soldiers with combat neurosis didn't rise again until the Vietnam War. So many of the men who fought in that war felt that they were doing so for no good reason. Never before had Americans been so openly divided about a war being fought by their soldiers. As the fighting ground on and on and the war came to an end without any clear winner or loser, the men who had been there exhibited signs of combat neurosis in huge numbers. Hundreds of "rap groups" were organized by veterans to give them a place to talk about their experiences. Because of the rising awareness of post-war trauma, post-traumatic stress syndrome was clearly defined and entered into the American Psychiatric Association's official diagnostic manual in the 1980s.

Feminism and Consciousness Raising

Right around the time Vietnam veterans were getting together to try to heal themselves, feminism was raising awareness of the incredible prevalence of rape and abuse—not only that which occurs between strangers, but between husbands and wives and between children and their older male relatives. Rather than trying to keep their personal problems quiet in order to avoid shaming themselves or breaking up their families, women began to feel that it was okay to speak out about the abuses and violence they had suffered. They found that people were willing to believe their stories because they were all so similar. So many women were telling the same ones about their own lives that to accuse them all of lying would have been impossible.

One study involving 900 randomly selected women revealed that one in three had been sexually abused in childhood, and that one in four had been raped. [Diana Russell] Feminism referred to this throwing open of the floodgates that had hidden abuse, rape, and domestic violence as *consciousness raising.* Psychologist Lenore Walker coined the phrase *battered woman syndrome* to describe the post-traumatic stress suffered by women who had been abused by their partners.

In 2000, the National Crime Victimization Survey reported that 249,000 people had been subjected to rape, attempted rape, or sexual assault. According to the NCVS, 44 percent of rape victims included in that survey were under the age of 18, and it was estimated that 15 percent of rape victims are under the age of 12. Two-thirds of those who commit rape are acquainted with or related to their victims. Fewer than 39 percent of sexual assaults are believed to be reported to law enforcement, and even those who do report sexual crimes against themselves are not likely to see their attacker punished. Only six percent of rapists end up in prison.

Clearly, consciousness raising has brought the problems of sexual and domestic violence to the world's attention, but we still have a long way to go.

A sizeable body of research indicates that the sexual abuse of children contributes powerfully to depression, addiction, chronic gastrointestinal disease, and suicide. Having been abused makes you more likely to abuse.

Inner City Trauma: A Meeting of the Minds

As early as 1970, the problem of trauma in children who live in the inner city has been recognized. Meers and Gordon: "Since traumatization is endemic in the ghetto…this might produce in the child some equivalent of 'combat fatigue.'" (Meers and Gordon, 1975.) Erwin Randolph Parson has given a name to this brand of traumatic stress syndrome: *urban violence traumatic stress syndrome* (U-VTS).

Today, no one with any real authority on the subject can deny the importance of childhood trauma in shaping the adults individuals become. Neither can they deny that in most cases, except in the most resilient of people, trauma leaves lasting marks on physical and psychological health, predisposing victims to illnesses of body and difficulties of spirit throughout their lifetimes. What is not widely acknowledged is the disproportionate effect childhood trauma has in the African-American community.

Most people know that proportionally, more crime is committed by African-Americans than other minorities or by Caucasians. Most people know that most of the faces that peer through the bars of prison cells are brown or black. The socioeconomic status of and educational opportunities for African-Americans are both less than those of Caucasians. Poorer blacks are more likely to live in crowded conditions in inner cities, where violence has come to be seen as a way of life. Six to twelve times as many African-Americans are victims of homicide in comparison with whites. Over the past three decades, the trend has been for increasing socioeconomic inequality—an ever-increasing gap between haves and have-nots—and for the concentration of poverty within minorities and within inner cities. (Kodras 1997; Lynn and McGeary 1990; Massey, Gross, and Eggers 1991; Wilson 1987.)

If we are to deal with the problem of violence—which is overwhelmingly concentrated in inner cities—we must address the traumas that are suffered by the children who live there. The cycle can only be broken with understanding, and understanding comes only from open-minded study and unfettered discourse.

The idea that inner-city children and the adults they become need help dealing with trauma is not a new one. My work builds on the work of other psychologists and psychiatrists, including Carl Bell, M.D., Bessel van der Kolk, Joy DeGruy-Leary, Gloria Johnson-Powell, M.D., and Stephen Kurtz. I will draw from the work of these thinkers and healers throughout the rest of these pages.

Stephen Kurtz began his work in Harlem in 1985. As a psychotherapist working in the South Bronx, he discovered that the people there had great "imagination, intelligence, and other gifts" that were going untapped because of extreme poverty and the physical and spiritual afflictions that come with it. He worked at a school in Harlem as a consultant psychotherapist, and found that the parents of the children he hoped to help were extremely wary of him. The children, on the other hand, were open to and in great need of his support—so much so that Dr. Kurtz opened the Harlem Family Institute in 1991. Children most needing therapy in the inner city are least likely to be part of families who can afford it, and the Institute was opened to serve these underserved and highly deserving young people. He continues to work to meet the needs of poor children for compassionate, effective psychotherapy.

Bessel van der Kolk is one of the world's most renowned minds when it comes to the modern-day study of psychological trauma. In his definitive textbook on the subject, *Traumatic Stress* (The Guilford Press, 1996), he states that "reenactment of victimization is a major cause of violence in society." Recognizing the truth of this statement is central to solving the problems of violence in the African-American community. Those who are victimized all too often desire to victimize others, in an effort to regain a sense of power and control. Perpetuating the vicious cycle of victimization does not heal the wounds that made the aggressor a victim in the first place.

Gloria Johnson Powell, M.D., is an expert on the role of culture in the psychology of children. She is the author of *The Psychosocial Development of Minority Group Children* and of *Transcultural Child Development: A Portrait of America's Children.* Her work aims to recognize and appreciate the impact of different cultural heritages on the ability of children to live healthy, fulfilled lives. She acknowledges that today's racism is much more complicated than black vs. white.

Joy DeGruy-Leary, PhD, was born in Los Angeles. She holds several degrees, including a doctorate in Social Work Research. Her twenty-plus years of social work have focused on teenaged and adult prostitutes, homeless children and young adults, and minority children and adults with chronic mental illness or who are at risk of developing mental illness. She counsels at-risk kids and teaches other counselors to help them stay in school and on the right track, rather than in gangs or involved in drug abuse, crime, or premature sexual activity. Dr. DeGruy-Leary also consults with organizations, educating people about cross-cultural sensitivity, human resource management in settings where more than one race works together, AIDS awareness, sexual harassment, and discrimination. Her culturally sensitive educational model for working with children and adults of color has been implemented in public schools in her home town of Portland, Oregon.

Dr. DeGruy-Leary has been the pioneering force in research into the intergenerational trauma that originated with slavery, which she calls Post-Traumatic Slave Syndrome. She has also created a psychological assessment instrument, called the African American Male Youth Respect Scale, designed to help keep young black men out of prison.

Carl Bell, M.D., likes to share a lesson he learned in medical school with those who attend his lectures or read his articles. The lesson is this: when a child with a rat bite walks into your clinic, you treat the rat bite with antibiotics, give the child a tetanus shot, and clean and dress the wound carefully, and that makes you a good doctor. But if 50 children with rat bites show up in need of treatment, you ought to lose your medical license if you do all of the above but don't go out into the community and do away with the rat. Since 1976, when he treated a four-year-old girl who had watched her mother get stabbed, Dr. Bell has worked tirelessly to try and kill off the rat—which is, in this case, violence.

In 1984, Dr. Bell surveyed 534 children, from the second to the eighth grade, in an inner-city setting. He found that a third of them had seen a shooting or stabbing. His next survey, this one of women who came to a community health clinic, he found that a third of them had been raped. Neither the staff at the clinic or the system they used to treat patients held any consciousness of the need for dealing with the impact of rape trauma (or any other kind of trauma) in these patients. In a 1989 survey, Dr. Bell found that of 1000 schoolchildren, 40 percent had seen a shooting, four percent had been stabbed, 10 percent had been shot, and 23 percent had witnessed a murder. A fourth study, performed in 1992 on 203 teenagers (aged 13 to 18) who lived in one of the most crime-ridden areas of Chicago, found that 60 percent of the children had seen a shooting, 45 percent had seen a stabbing, and 43 percent had seen a murder.

In the course of his research, Dr. Bell made some important observations. Freud and Breuer, he observed, had worked with grown women; not much research had been done on how to help small children to process and overcome traumatic events and PTSD. He saw that: children who had been traumatized once were more likely to suffer from post-traumatic stress and anxiety, while those who were under chronic stress that continually traumatized them were more prone to behavioral problems and academic underachievement; sexual assault in female children made them much more likely to abuse drugs as adults; a child who is hypervigilant because of trauma is not going to be able to learn in school; a child who is traumatized at a very young age—let's say, by sexual abuse—she is likely to be retraumatized as she grows older and recognizes the full depth and breadth of what happened to her.

Once he had a grasp of the problem, Dr. Bell began to work on solutions. His research has revealed factors that reduce the impact of traumatic stress on children, including good parenting during infancy, a strong family and community support system, and a quality he calls *resiliency*—a combination of characteristics that enables human beings to surmount whatever fate throws their way. Dr. Bell was one of the first trauma specialists to integrate holistic health principles, including traditional Chinese medicine, t'ai chi, chi kung, and breath work, into trauma therapy.

Current research indicates that the effects of trauma become "hard-wired" into the brain by the time a traumatic event is two days past. It also has been found that this hard-wiring can be prevented if the right interventions are made within that two-day window. Dr. Bell formed the American Academy of Pediatrics Task Force on Assault Victims Needs to try to get emergency room staff the training they need to help trauma victims as soon as they reach the hospital.

The Next Step

If you put too many rats in a single cage, they begin to do violence to one another, and the same thing happens with human beings in crowded cities, suburbs, and schools. It doesn't *have* to happen, however. People are capable of organizing and cooperating in ways that rats are not. We are capable of understanding, supporting, and helping one another. We are capable of forgiveness and empathy.

History has made clear the need for two gifts we need to offer to children at risk for psychological trauma. First, we must develop effective ways to help them heal once they have suffered a traumatic event. Second, we must do what we can to understand the roots of that event and the basis upon which they react to it, and we must use that understanding to protect children from the harm trauma can do.

Chapter Three

Community Trauma and Post-Traumatic Slave Syndrome

Trauma links past to present through representations and imagination.
—Maya Angelou

The personal meaning of traumatic experience for individuals is influenced by the social context in which it occurs. Victims and the significant people in their surroundings may have different and fluctuating assessments of both the reality of what has happened and of the extent of the victims' suffering. As a result, victims and bystanders may have strongly conflicting agendas to repair, create, forget, or take revenge. These conflicts between the victims' and the bystanders' assessment of the meaning of the trauma may set the stage for the trauma to be perpetuated in a larger social setting; soon the allocation of blame and responsibility, not the trauma itself, may become the central issue.
—Alexander McFarlane and Bessel Van der Kolk, *Traumatic Stress,* p. 26-27.

Post-traumatic slave syndrome is a topic that raises controversy wherever I bring it up. Some assume that by labeling the problems of today's African-Americans as an outgrowth of slavery, I am suggesting that the descendants of those who were traumatized by slavery are entitled to reparations or other special privileges, or that bad behavior on the part of African-Americans should be forgiven because of the history of their race.

Let me say up front that I am not for or against reparations. My concern with post-traumatic slave syndrome is not about making excuses for bad behavior, or about money. It is about healing. I believe that acknowledging the impact of the nightmare of slavery on the African-American race is an important part of the healing process for these people. We need to heal from that community tragedy. Failure to do so will impede our healing from the other ills that afflict us.

Others say that Africans were not the only enslaved people, and that most races have been subjugated at some time in history. If virtually everyone has been traumatized by enslavement or prejudice, what good could I possibly be doing as I single out African-American post-traumatic stress?

Again, let me say that I don't wish to give African-American issues any more weight than Irish-American, Muslim-American, or Asian-American issues. But the facts are the facts: blacks in America do more of the crime and more of the time than anyone in any other racial group, and they disproportionately inhabit the lower rungs of the economic ladder. When a child acts out and, in so doing, hurts himself and others, he is showing those around him that he needs more attention, more tenderness, more support, and a chance to heal. On a larger scale, this is the message coming loud and clear from the African-American community. I hope that by shining a light on the need for healing from post-slavery trauma, I will also illuminate the need for other races to process and heal from the traumas that have affected their predecessors.

Traumas like slavery, the Holocaust, and the wholesale destruction of Native American tribes affect entire races of people, and they affect the ways in which these people parent their children, and their children parent their own children, and so on. This is one way in which trauma is perpetuated through generations.

An acquaintance of mine is a fourth-generation Jewish American. This is what she told me when we discussed the concept of cultural trauma:

Since I was a small child, my parents talked about the Holocaust. None of our family went through it, but it was a huge part of our consciousness. I remember lying on the floor looking through books, staring at photographs of emaciated prisoners, reading about the atrocities and just being blown away by it all. I never thought about it until now, but I can definitely see how the consciousness of those millions of Jews being persecuted affected the way my parents parented me. They were overprotective—smotheringly so. I learned from them that the world is a very, very dangerous place. And they absolutely insisted that I put on a happy face, no matter what. No negativity was allowed to come up. If you felt bad, you had to take it somewhere else. It was as if they were saying, "Don't you know you're lucky to even be alive, to be free from persecution? How dare *you complain about anything!" And I can see how all of this has affected the way I parent my own children.*

An African-American patient with grown sons told me:

It's sad, what's going on with our young people. My sons didn't learn how to be men. Real men who can take care of their own, I mean. They have all the right equipment for making babies, and they've done that, but they're not doing what they should to take care of those babies. I keep asking myself what I did wrong raising them. Was it that they didn't have a daddy to show them the way? Probably, that was part of it. But then I think about how I coddled them and spoiled them and didn't make them take responsibility. I felt like the world is going to be such a hard place for them as black people, I wanted them to have it easy at least for a little while, at home with their mamma.

There is more to community trauma than its effect on parenting. In his book *Cultural Trauma: Slavery and the Formation of African-American History* (Cambridge Press, 2001), Ron Eyerman describes community trauma as an event that tears the social fabric of a cohesive group of people, causing a dramatic loss of identity and meaning. Whether the loss happened yesterday or a generation ago, the struggle to reestablish identity and meaning continues until they are found or until the group disbands entirely. This can happen in the span of a few years, or of a few lifetimes, or of centuries.

The identity of an individual is built on the foundation of her past. That past is almost always a collectively remembered history, shared between family members and friends. That history may be acknowledged from time to time by the larger community of humanity; for example, by memorials to those who have fought in wars, or by the information included in history books. No matter how carefully a record is made of the past, it is colored by the interpretations of those who record it and report it. Those who were actually involved in the happening being described—for example, for the footsoldiers in the Vietnam war—have a different experience than do those who observed it, perhaps as medics or journalists or civilians who saw the carnage but did not directly participate in it. If you were to ask a number of people who were present at or involved in a traumatic episode, you would hear stories that varied so much that you'd wonder if everyone really experienced the same thing. Interpretations of the past are often affected by the present needs of the people who are doing the interpreting.

To quote a phrase often used when feminism burst into the mainstream, *the personal is political.* The self develops within the context of a social framework, and that framework shapes the development of the self. Social frameworks develop over generations. It follows that a trauma that affected an entire race and culture a century or more ago would continue to affect the children of those who were initially traumatized, and their children's children, and so on down to the children being born today.

Slavery in America

The institution of slavery has existed at least since 3500 B.C., when the ancient Egyptians enslaved those who were taken as prisoners of war. The prosperity of ancient Greece and Rome were built upon the backs of slaves. Early Europeans and Africans also engaged in the practice of keeping slaves as servants, artisans, and laborers. By the 11th century, Muslim traders were capturing natives in North Africa and selling them to other Islamic countries. Even then, it became evident that Negroes made the best slaves: they were strong, and their skin color made them easy to differentiate from their captors.

Between the 16th and 19th centuries, the trade in African men, women, and children to and from the New World far surpassed any other system of slavery, both in its cruelty and its enormity. More than eleven million Africans—and some say that this estimate is much lower than the true number of black and brown people forced to migrate to North America—were shipped across the sea in the holds of jam-packed slave boats to endure forced servitude in the newly forming nation.

In 1640, Maryland became the first state to institutionalize slavery. By 1750, over 200,000 slaves toiled in the fields, homes, workshops, and factories of America. In Virginia alone, three-fourths of the families owned slaves, and they were being imported into the state at the rate of 1,000 per year by 1700. By 1800, the number of slaves living in America topped 700,000—about one-sixth of the population of the so-called "land of the free." By 1830, the slave population in the South had reached two million.

It is no exaggeration to say that much of the current wealth of America was built on the whip-scarred backs of slaves. Without the work they did in the early years of American farming, plantation owners never would have been able to prosper as they did.

Slave trade became illegal in the U.S. in 1808—not because it was unethical, but because Americans feared that slaves would revolt if their population surpassed that of the whites. Still, a very profitable black-market slave trade continued well past the Emancipation Proclamation, made in 1863. Slaveholders were eager to profit from interstate sales of slaves to newly forming states such as Mississippi, Alabama, and Texas, and they pushed their slaves to reproduce as quickly as possible, often trying to arrange matches that they believed would produce the hardiest children*:

Master would sometimes go and get a large, hale, hearty Negro man from some other plantation to go to his Negro woman. He would ask the other master to let this man come over to his place to

*All of the quotes from ex-slaves in this chapter have been taken, unless otherwise specified, from Bullwhip Days: The Slaves Remember, An Oral History (James Mellon, ed.; Weidenfield and Nicolson, New York, NY: 1988.) This book is a collection of narratives gathered during interviews with ex-slaves in the 1930s during the Works Progress Administration.

go to his slave girls. A slave girl was expected to have children as soon as she became a woman. Some of them had children at the age of twelve and thirteen years old. Negro men six feet tall went to some of these children.

—Hilliard Yellerday

Children born to slaves were the property of the owner of their mother. With one man fathering children by several women, fathers were often not a part of family life in slave communities. This is where today's problems with absent fathers in the African-American community began. Slave owners often "used" slave women as mistresses, and it was not unusual for these white men's children to be born into slavery. One ex-slave told of refusing her master's advances and being forced to sit naked on a pile of manure until she gave in.

Babies and young children were usually cared for by an older slave woman who could no longer work in the fields. Some owners did not allow mothers adequate time for visiting their infants to nurse them or care for them, and many babies ended up dying from the lack of attention. Despite the hard conditions they found themselves under, many slave women ended up giving birth to eight, ten, thirteen children. Many had to watch most of those children sold away to other masters long before they were ready to do without their mothers.

Slave codes designated that slaves were not people, and that they were property that could be sold at any time. Slaves were not allowed to marry, have gatherings (unless permission was given by the master), hit a white person (even in self-defense), or leave their homes or plantations without permission given in writing. They were not allowed to visit or be visited by whites or free blacks, or to learn to read or write.

Even so, slave culture was rich with song and dance, and weekends and Christmastime were, for some slaves, filled with fun and social activity. Some slaves had better situations than others. Not all masters were cruel; many provided their slaves with plenty of food, adequate shelter, and did all they could to keep their slaves happy. Others worked their slaves to the bone, giving them barely enough food to survive and whipping them for the slightest infraction.

Ise sho' 'joy myse'f on de old plantation, an' we-uns all had a good time. Allus have plenty to eat. Marster used to say, 'De cullud folks raised de food, an' dey's 'titled to all dey wants.' Same wid de clothes.

—Florence Napier

De nigger used to sing to nearly everything he did. Hit wuz jes' de way he 'spressed his feelin's, an' hit made him relieved. If he wuz happy, hit made him happier; if he wuz sad, hit made him feel better. An' so, he jes' naturally sings his feelin's...Singin' is de niggers' mos' joy an' dey mos' comfort. When dey needs all dese things, dey sing 'bout de joys in de nex' world an' de trouble in dis.

—Vinnie Brunson

The place of song and dance in today's African-American communities was firmly established by those long, hard days of slave labor.

No textbook facts can adequately reflect the details of the degradation many slaves were forced to endure. Africans who had been kidnapped or given into slavery (some African nations sold lawbreakers to slave traders) often were brought to the coast in forced marches that resulted in the deaths of millions. All along the west coast of Africa, slaveholding sites built by Europeans were used to house those destined for slave ships. Those awaiting sale to slave traders were put to work and packed into nearly airless cells at night with dozens of others.

For those who survived the trip to the coast, there was the horrifying ordeal of the slave ships, where men, women, and children were chained to one another, hand to hand and foot to foot or by the neck, stacked together like firewood. Imagine the horror of being captured—either by white slave traders or by an opposing army in a war in your own land—and loaded onto a ship for a long journey, not knowing where you are going or what awaits you when you arrive. The journey took from five to 12 weeks. About 13 percent of the 12 or 13 million Africans shipped overseas as slaves died during the voyage. Some leapt off of the ships to drown in the ocean rather than face a horrifying present and an uncertain future.

The ones that survived the journey to the New World were sold, usually at auction. Slaves were an expensive investment, but one that paid off over the long haul. A strong, healthy young man could go for as much as $2,500 to $2,800, while a small child would set a colonist back about $250. Families were routinely split apart and sold to different masters, never to see one another again.

Man, man, folks what didn't go through slavery ain't got no idea what it was. I reckon there musta been a hundred colored folks in that trader yard, and the dirt and smell was terrible, terrible. I was jes' a little chap, like I've told you, but I can remember that place like it happened yesterday—husbands sold away from wives, and children taken away from mothers. A trader, them days, didn't think no more of selling a baby or little child away from its mother than taking a little calf away from a cow.

—Stephen Williams

The bidders have white gloves there, and one of the bidders takes a pair of gloves and rubs his fingers over a man's teeth, and he says to the overseer, "You call this buck twenty years old? Why there's cup worms in his teeth. He's forty years old, if he's a day." So they knock this buck down for a thousand dollars. They calls the men 'bucks' and the women 'wenches.'

...At these slave auctions, the overseer yells, "Say, you bucks and wenches, get in your hole. Come out here." Then, he makes 'em hop, he makes 'em trot, he makes 'em jump.

—James Martin

Many of the more benevolent masters manipulated their slaves into obedience by telling them how bad things were for slaves on other plantations.

If one slave kilt another, Marse Billy made de overseer tie dat dead nigger to de one what kilt him, and de killer had to drag de corpse round till he died, too. De murderers never lived long a-draggin' them dead ones round. Dat jus' piorely skeered 'em to death.

—Callie Elder

Folks a mile away could hear dem awful whippings. Dey wuz a turrible part of livin'.
—Delia Garlic

My moster would put slaves in a calaboose at night to be whipped de next morning. He always limited de lashes to five hundred. After whipping dem, he would rub pepper and salt on deir backs, where whipped, and lay dem before de fire until blistered, and den take a cat, and hold de cat, and make him claw de blisters, to burst dem.
—Robert Burns

My husband said there was a family named Gullendin which was mighty hard on their niggers. He said ole Missis Gullendin, she'd take a needle and stick it through one of their nigger women's lower lip and pin it to the bosom of her dress, and the woman would go roun' all day with her haid drew down thataway, and slobberin'. Ole Missis Gullendin done her that-away lots of times. There was knots on her lip where the needle had been stuck in it. Me, I don't b'lieve I coulda stood that no time, without goin' crazy.
—Mrs. Thomas Johns

Masters rarely killed slaves outright. They were valuable property. Their punishments and mistreatments were designed to impose as much suffering and fear as possible without hampering their ability to recover and go back to work.

Plantation work was backbreaking. Slaves were flogged for not doing as much as their white overseers believed they could. According to the record of a slave named Henry Bibb, "some overseers…instituted so-called contests in which the slave in each group who picked the most cotton would receive the equivalent of a dollar or two in valuables. 'After making them try it over several times and weighing what cotton they pick every night, the overseer can tell just how much every hand can pick,' Bibb recounted. 'He then gives the present to those that pick the most cotton, and then if they do not pick just as much afterward they are flogged.'" [from *African-American Voices of Triumph: Perseverance,* Time-Life Books, Alexandria VA: 1993, page 33]

Children were often put to work by the time they were five or six years old. Slaves usually lived in poorly built one—to two-room cabins, with as many as 12 people crammed in when it finally came time to go to sleep at night. They sweltered in the summer and froze in the winter.

This is not to say that slaves by and large accepted their lot and lived out their lives trying to serve their masters as best they could. There are many inspiring stories of slaves revolting against their chains, in ways big and small:

We stole so many chickens that if a chicken would see a darkey he'd run right straight to the house.

—Anonymous

My mother, she didn't work in the field. She worked at a loom. She worked so long and so often that once she went to sleep at the loom. Her master's boy saw her and told his mother. His mother told him to take a whip and wear her out. He took a stick and went out to beat her awake. He beat my mother till she woke up. When she woke up, she took a pole out of the loom and beat him nearly to death with it. He hollered, 'Don't beat me no more, and I won't let 'em whip you.' She said, 'I'm goin' to kill you. These black titties sucked you, and then you come out here to beat me.' And when she left him, he wasn't able to walk.

And that was the last I seen of her until after Freedom. She went and got an old cow she used to milk—Dolly, she called it. She rode away from the plantation, because she knew they would kill her, if she stayed.

—Ellen Cragin

Old Mistress got sick, and I would fan her with a brush, to keep the flies off her. I would hit her all in the face. Sometimes, I would make out I was asleep and beat her in the face. She was so sick she couldn't sleep much, and couldn't talk, and when Old Master come in the house, she would try to tell him on me, but he thought she just meant I would go to sleep. Then, he would tell me to go out in the yard and wake up. She couldn't tell him that I had been hitting her all in the face. I done that woman bad. She was so mean to me.

—Anonymous

Slaves would also work slowly, pretend not to understand instructions, break tools, kill livestock, set fires. White slave-owners attributed these problems to the inferior intelligence of their slaves.

A few slave revolts took place, including the one orchestrated by Nat Turner and by Gabriel Prosser in Virginia. The revolt of Africans on the ship *Amistad* and the trial that followed was one of the few successful slave revolts; the story was made into a film by Steven Spielberg. Most revolts were short-lived and led to the deaths of many freedom-seeking slaves. Following some of the revolts, the white men who had quashed them would cut the heads off of the dead revolutionaries and impale them on posts along the roadside, as a warning to others who had the same ideas.

Many slaves also were able to escape their masters. Some escaped slaves went up North via the Underground Railroad. Others slipped into the swamplands of the South, forming communities of fugitives—also called *maroons,* an Anglicized version of the Spanish word *cimarrón,* which translates to *wild.* Around 50 such communities existed in the wilderness.

Slavery and the African-American Identity

The African-American identity was created, in significant part, by the reality of slavery. Even blacks who never lived under slavery—those who arrived in the New World as free men and who were central to efforts to free their African-American brothers and sisters—were affected by the knowledge that at any time, they could be thrown into chains and sold into slavery because of the color of their skin. This happened to many freedmen before the Emancipation.

Whether a slave's existence was better or worse than that of the average slave, his situation was a traumatic one. He was helpless, his life completely dictated by factors outside of his control. In some instances, slaves were in constant fear of beatings or death, and had to watched loved ones suffer the same fear and helplessness without any way of coming to their aid. Living under these kinds of circumstances quickly breaks a person's spirit, teaches her to put away her feelings and try to eke the best possible life from the ruins she finds herself in. Comfort was found within the tight bonds forged within the slave community, within song, within small acts of rebellion.

Ron Eyerman writes that the "trauma of forced servitude came to be central to attempts…to forge a collective identity." One of the best ways to drive human beings to bond together and forge this kind of collective identity is to make them slaves.

It is true that some African-Americans were able to prosper while others were enslaved. Records show that in New Orleans in the year 1860, approximately 18,000 free blacks owned $15 million worth of property. In fact, many wealthy African-Americans owned black slaves themselves. Some black slaveowners bought their relatives as slaves to circumvent laws mandating that newly freed slaves must leave the place where they had once been owned as property; in some cases, slaves owned by African-Americans were used for the same purposes as those owned by whites.

Slaves who reported being treated well and having genuine affection for their masters may have had it better than other slaves, but they were still slaves who could be bought, sold, or beaten at any time. Trauma literature describes the Stockholm syndrome, where prisoners grow to sympathize with and even love their captors. Being so dependent upon the person who holds one captive inspires gratitude in the person being held prisoner. The smallest kindnesses feel like huge generosity to those who are enslaved and subjugated.

The Struggles of New Freedom

On April 9, 1865, the Conferedate army surrendered. From that point forward, Confederate states acknowledged that they had no rights to own black people or force them into servitude. Once the slaves were freed, they went out into the world to try to find work, find homes, and raise their families in a nation that still believed them to be an inferior race that did not have the rights white people enjoyed.

Over the next 12 years—a period known as the Reconstruction—a nation torn apart by civil war worked to rebuild itself. The government put into place the Bureau of Freedmen, Refugees, and Abandoned Lands to help newly freed slaves make the transition into free life.

Some newly freed slaves rejoiced; others were reluctant to leave homes that were secure and masters who had been good to them.

I think slavery wus good, because I was treated all right. I think I am 'bout as much a slave now, as ever. 'Bout half the folks, both black an' white, is slaves an' don't know it.

—Jerry Hinton

Everybody wants to be free, and they should be. I don't believe it's right to live in bondage, but I do say it bold and aboveboard that the slaves with good masters, like mine, was a heap better off. I can remember having everything I wanted, and it takes a long time to get used to not having nothing.

—Mark Oliver

Food and clothing were scarce in the South during the winter after the Civil War. The Freedmen's Bureau tried to help out by delivering rations to those most in need. But, as the old saying goes, give a man a fish and he eats for one day; teach a man how to fish and he'll have food for the rest of his life. The freed African-Americans knew how to work hard, but they didn't have the skills they needed to thrive in a world that seemed to revolve around money. Many freed slaves had never even seen money before they were set free.

Many freedmen were forced into sharecropping, where they were given a piece of land on a plantation and a line of credit (to buy supplies and food from the plantation owner) in return for part of the profits made on their crops. It was rare for any of these sharecroppers to come out ahead. With the interest charged on their credit and high prices for the things they bought with that credit, sharecroppers struggled to break even.

Under the Southern Homestead Act, 4,000 blacks who had been loyal to the Union cause were given 80 acres and a startup grant in either Alabama, Arkansas, Florida, Louisiana, or Mississippi. Most of these farms failed because the land was poor and whites in those areas were hardly welcoming. All in all, freedmen worked as hard as they had under slavery, and ended up with little or nothing to show for it.

Socioeconomic inequality is a traumatic state of affairs, and this inequality still affects African-Americans. When entire segments of society feel they have been unjustly treated, when they feel cut off from comfort and plenty, when they feel mired in poverty and have no hope for a better life, this is traumatic in and of itself.

Andrew Johnson became President, and instituted laws that eliminated African-Americans from government and judicial processes. Congress opposed this trend by ratifying the 14th Amendment, which dictated that anyone born in the U.S.—black or white (but, interestingly, not Native American)—would be a citizen and would have the right to vote. Little by little over the next 100 years, the U.S. government changed government to include African-Americans as the equals of whites.

Ninety-seven percent of African-Americans did not know how to read or write at the end of the Civil War. Over 4,000 schools were created to educate blacks who craved knowledge after long years of being kept ignorant under slavery. When it came time to integrate white and black children in Southern public schools—which didn't happen until nearly 1960—it took armed soldiers to preserve the peace. Segregated drinking fountains, public transportation, and restaurants provoked African-Americans into legal challenges and sit-ins that eventually overcame attempts to keep them separated from whites. The peaceful war waged by Martin Luther King, Jr. helped unify African-Americans, brought their plight into the public eye, and brought many supportive whites into the civil rights struggle, but his assassination took him from his cause much too soon. Most people alive today have some grasp of this part of American history.

The scars from the prejudicial treatment African-Americans have suffered run deep. Being consistently devalued, prejudiced against, insulted, and subjugated; being treated unfairly by the legal system—all of the injustices suffered by blacks at the hands of those who believed that they were fundamentally inferior—perpetuated the wounds left by slavery. As a culture, African-Americans are re-traumatized by these kinds of injustices. Thousands of black men (and a few women) were lynched in the years following emancipation, many for little more than saying the wrong thing within earshot of a racist with violent tendencies. According to the Tuskeegee Institute in Alabama, the last black person to fall prey to a lynch mob was the 4,742nd one who had met this fate since 1882. Believe it or not, this lynching happened in 1964.

Today, black men are the object of more hatred and fear than most whites are willing to admit. They are stereotyped as dangerous criminals because of the color of their skin. One white colleague admitted to me that

...although I know that a black person isn't, by nature, any more dangerous than a white person, I still feel afraid when I spot a black man coming towards me. I hate it that I feel that fearfulness. I like to think of myself as progressive, the opposite of racist, open to people of all races. But I can't seem to stop that fear response from coming up.

White men came to this country and decimated the peaceful Native American cultures they found and took their land. Then, they began to keep Africans in bondage. Predominantly white America has a long history of other insults against other races and cultures, and they have predominated over those races and cultures primarily through the use of brute force. And still, the black man is the object of our fear and hatred. Why?

Think of the typical bully. He's on a rampage, picking on everyone, making a lot of people's lives miserable. Eventually, he's going to get his comeuppance. Someone is going to beat the tar out of him, or he's going to get kicked out of school, or some other terrible thing is going to happen to him. Knowing this—knowing that having threatened others, he himself is under threat—he escalates his bullying. He lives in a constant state of fear and anger. He does worse and worse deeds to those around him. He picks on those least able to defend themselves.

When blacks became free, whites feared that those who once were their prisoners would turn around and—as the expression goes—open up a big can of whoop-ass. They did not. It seems, sometimes, that the whites are still waiting, terrified, for the revolution.

It is also the case that once subjugated people become free, they tend to try to subjugate others. Remember that most of the violence done to black people is done by other blacks.

Chapter Four

Why Children Turn Violent

A society functions as a reflection of its childrearing practices. If children are ignored, poorly educated and not protected from violence, they will grow into adults that create a reactive, non-creative and violent society...All societies reap what they have sown.

—Bruce Perry, "The Neurodevelopmental Impact of Violence in Childhood," in *Textbook of Child and Adolescent Forensic Psychiatry,* Schetky and Benedek, editors; American Psychiatric Press, Inc., Washington, DC.

Gang violence, school shootings, and garden-variety bullying and tormenting in schools and around the neighborhoods are all on the rise. One child murders another because he wants that child's cool new sneakers. Other children and teenagers claim that their violent acts were done in self-defense, or in defense of their gang, or to protect their reputations. Many only seem remorseful about having been caught.

Some violence done by children is the result of a dangerous combination of the influence of violent heroes in the media with inadequate self-control, as was likely the case with the 12-year-old boy who killed a six-year-old playmate while imitating pro wrestling moves he'd seen on television. In some cases, child murderers take their own lives rather than face the consequences of what they have done. Others doom themselves to a life behind bars.

I took a life, an innocent life when I come to really think about it. I had to do it or be kicked off the set [gang]. *I had to prove that I was down. I had to show everybody that I was hardcore...He called me Blood, a name that I ain't supposed to like. He challenged my dedication to my 'hood and disrespected my dead homeboys. "Kill that fool," one of my homeboys yelled. I pulled out my best friend, aimed it at his head, closed my eyes, and squeezed the trigger one time. I heard his body fall to the concrete...I watched as blood hid his entire face.*

—Aaron Collins, *The Gangbanger,* reprinted in *Gangs: Opposing Viewpoints,* David Bender and Bruno Leone, Series Eds., Charles P. Cozick, Book Ed., Greenhaven Press, San Diego CA: 1996.

The violence done to children isn't only done by other children, of course. Adults harm children far more, both intentionally and unintentionally. It could be argued that children hurt themselves just as often—through behaviors such as self-mutilation, attempts at suicide, or through other self-destructive behaviors where they put themselves in harm's way again and again. Examples that come to mind are girls who repeatedly get involved with abusive boys or men, and children who abuse alcohol and drugs.

The sources of violence against children vary widely, but fortunately for those of us who wish to stop such violence, the causes are almost always the same. *Children kill or harm others, or kill or harm themselves, because of traumas they have suffered, sometimes beginning from their first day on this earth.* The impact of trauma on children can damage them both physically and psychologically during pivotal points in their development, especially if that trauma is chronic—occurring repeatedly over an extended period of time.

When a developmental stage is disrupted because of trauma, the stages that follow are disrupted as well. This is akin to putting too much sand in the cement when building the foundation of a house: it might hold together for a while, but it will begin to crumble. Eventually, your house is going to start to crumble, and if a big storm comes along it's more likely to topple. Or, sometimes, a child gets stuck in the developmental stage during which the trauma occurred or began, and never grows up.

Types of Violence

Many kinds of violence affect children of all races and in all levels of socioeconomic status. These different kinds of violence can have dramatically different effects on children.

Violence against children is not a singularly African-American problem; it isn't even a mostly African-American problem. Most evidence shows us that the problems of child violence and child abuse belong to people of every color. There is, however, a much greater problem with *community violence* in the African-American culture—the inner cities where five shootings of young black people can happen in a single weekend. Examples of community violence are gang warfare and rioting.

A child who lives and goes to school in a bad neighborhood lives in constant fear. He may see others shot, stabbed, or attacked on a regular basis.

It has been estimated that at least half of inner-city children have witnessed violent acts—stabbings, shootings, murders, beatings, rapes. Many of these violent acts occur in the child's home, between people the child depends upon and loves. It is difficult to overestimate the damage this does to a young child.

Domestic violence includes violence done between adults as well as child abuse. At least five million American children are victims of or witnesses to domestic violence, physical abuse, or community violence. According to an FBI report, 27 percent of all violent crime done in 1995 was inflicted by one family member on another, and 48 percent of violent crime was the result of an acquaintance doing violence on someone in his or her home. While these numbers are shocking, keep in mind that it's estimated that less than five percent of all incidences of domestic violence end up being reported.

Community and domestic violence can be *impulsive, predatory,* or *defensive.* Impulsive violence is the product of a combination of hyperarousal and decreased impulse control; a child might hit a classmate for putting his hand on the child's property, or a teenager might shoot a passerby because he believes him to be from a rival gang, or a parent might beat her young child because she can't control her anger at his naturally childish behaviors. Predatory violence is just what it sounds like: an angry, traumatized person violently preys on others—often because he feels threatened himself. Defensive violence is also just what it sounds like. I can't count the number of times a teenager in jail for murder has told me, "I had to do him before he did me," or "It was him or me," or some other variation on this theme.

Then, there's the added influence of violent television, movies, and computer games. The average 18-year-old has viewed 200,000 acts of violence on television. This may not be a direct cause of violence in children, but it certainly contributes. It sets forth violent heroes who become powerful and accomplished through the use of violence. The child who sees someone successfully using violence to get what he wants—whether in the home or on the small or big screen—is more likely to turn to violence when he himself feels powerless.

Neglect is a powerful part of the child trauma equation. In fact, neglect is one of the most insidious and ultimately harmful forms of child abuse. A child that is properly attended to can recover from other traumas, but a neglected child is left without coping mechanisms. Even children who seem to have it all—financial security, all the toys they could want, the latest fashions, a nice big house—can end up being neglected when parents substitute material things for their own time, love, and attention. The results of neglect can devastate a child, and neglectful homes are often homes where other risks to children exist: the threat of physical harm, persistent fear, and chaotic environments.

The Question (and Answer) of Blame

Before I move further into this topic, let me explain as clearly as I can that I do not wish to place blame here, and it's not my role as healer to decide who ought to get punished for the wrongs done to children. It is my role to awaken awareness—a truthful, no-holds-barred kind of awareness. It may sound like blaming from time to time, but this is not my intention. I know that many parents whose children turn to violence have done the best they possibly could—especially inner-city African-American women who were forced to raise their children alone, while holding a job and trying to eke out some small corner of life where they could feel fulfilled. They may have been trapped in an environment where their children were exposed to traumatic situations, no matter how hard their families tried to protect them.

I believe that without clear awareness of the sources of childhood trauma, there can be no healing. I also believe that for every parent who has done wrong by a child, there is another parent or family member further up the generations that perpetrated traumas on that parent. This is an intergenerational process. Perpetrators are victims, too. And let's not forget the fact that parenting is difficult even under the best of circumstances.

Taking blame is a very different thing from taking responsibility. If we are to heal America's children, we have all got to acknowledge what's hurting them. As Carl Bell would say, we must kill the rat that's biting our children.

I don't blame the individual parents for child violence. If I had to blame something, it would be the socioeconomic hierarchy that subjugates so many and lifts up so few. Those who are lifted up, for the most part, don't much care what's happening to those who are being downtrodden—until they feel threatened by the violence that once was only known by those living in the inner city. In the words of Tim Wise, a Nashville, Tennessee-based writer and activist:

> *What went wrong is that white Americans decided to ignore dysfunction and violence when it only affected other communities, and thereby blinded themselves to the inevitable creeping of chaos, which never remains isolated too long. What affects the urban 'ghetto' today will be coming to a Wal-Mart near you tomorrow, and unless you address the emptiness, pain, isolation and lack of hope felt by children of color and the poor, then don't be shocked when the support systems aren't there for your kids either.*
>
> —Tim Wise, "School Shootings and White Denial," *AlterNet*, http://www.alternet.com, March 6, 2001.

Traumatic experiences within the home and outside of the home can have very different effects on a child's development. If a child has a strong home base with parents who do all the right things, she is better equipped to handle the threat of violence outside of that home base. If she isn't parented well—and this can mean simply not having enough time or support from parents who are struggling to make ends meet—her risk of being damaged by community violence increases.

The link between child violence and more affluent, predominantly white areas is, of course, school shootings. These are not examples of inner-city violence or black violence—in fact, white children are twice as likely to bring a weapon to school than black children—but white suburban violence.

When a (white) child brings a gun to school and shoots a few of his classmates and teachers, the papers and the nightly news are filled with the story. Black-on-black violence doesn't get nearly as much air time. Why?

Well, the subtext goes something like this: *We expect black people to kill each other, but when a white child from a 'good home' in small-town America does something like this, it's a great big mystery.* I argue that it's no mystery at all. It all goes back to trauma. Neglect is an important but widely unacknowledged form of trauma, and it could be said that many children growing up in the suburbs are neglected by overworked, overscheduled parents and overcrowded schools. So is relentless teasing—the kind that the Columbine shooters suffered. As you'll read on, you'll find that trauma comes in many forms, and that the effects of trauma can begin to alter a child's development from the day of her birth forward.

Nature and Nurture in Traumatized Children

Some have argued that genetics dictate a person's violent tendencies; others, that the environment during childhood is to blame when an individual turns violent. Of course, a combination of these factors—nature and nurture—come into play.

Only a small minority of children become violent. Even those raised in neglectful or abusive situations are not likely to end up hurting others. The wounds are still there, but they show up in different forms: persistent depression, anxiety, a feeling of emptiness, difficulty relating to others, underachievement. All of these manifestations of childhood trauma contribute to the overall problem of violence, however. They affect the way children are parented. They affect socioeconomic status. They help to create an environment that breeds violence in that small group of children that ends up striking out at others.

Traumatic experience in childhood has direct effects on development. When an infant is born, it is completely dependent upon its caregivers. Neglect, poor parenting, or exposure to violence in infancy can damage a child for life.

- Historical information and scientific research show us how neglect can alter a child's biology, even to the point of causing children to give up on this life entirely:
- In the days of slavery, mothers who could not attend to their babies would be forced to hang them in slings of fabric from the branches of trees, returning to them only as often as they were allowed to by their masters. Many babies simply died from the lack of attention.
- Experiments with rhesus monkeys have repeatedly shown that baby monkeys raised without attention or stimulation develop violent tendencies towards others and themselves, engaging in head-banging, compulsive rocking, and other forms of self-injury.
- A study by Pollard and Perry demonstrated that of 12 children who experienced severe neglect, cortical atrophy—literally, shrinkage of the cortical brain—was found in seven.
- Rats raised in environmentally rich settings have 30 percent greater synaptic density, meaning that their brain cells are more interconnected.
- Animals raised in the wild—where their environments are rich and diverse— have 15 to 30 percent greater brain mass than their domestic cousins, who do not learn how to hunt, or how to socialize within a pack, or otherwise live the life a canine or feline creature is designed to live.
- Orphans who receive little to no individual attention as children often are damaged beyond repair. Their brain development lags far behind that of normal children.

Babies only know how to do one thing when they need attention or are afraid of something: they cry. A newborn's cry is custom-designed by nature to bring adults running so that the baby's needs can be attended to. When parents don't respond to a baby's cry consistently, two terrible things happen. First, the baby learns right away that its needs are not going to be met. Its signals are not being heeded. The baby stops trying, falling into a state known in psychology as *learned helplessness.* Second, the parent who is, for whatever reason, not responding to the infant's cry ends up not having a strong attachment to her baby. She overrides her instinctive need to respond to her baby's needs, and the instinct is pushed out of her awareness. Right away, she becomes less able to parent in a caring and nurturing way.

A baby who has learned that he cannot get the care he needs may become passive and compliant. He learns not to feel pain. He learns heartbreakingly early that the gratification of his needs is not something he can depend upon. As that child grows older, he is unable to conceive of a future, or of delayed gratification; he learns that if he wants something, he'd better grab onto it right now. The notion that behaviors have natural consequences also goes out the window in the neglected child.

Both emotional and physical abuse—two sides of the same coin—have dramatic effects on a child's developing brain. When a child first comes into the world, his brain still has a lot of growing and changing to do.

For our purposes, let's divide the brain into two distinct parts: the *limbic* brain and the *cortex*. At birth, the limbic brain—that part of the brain that manages basic body functions and drives—predominates. The cortex is responsible for reason, impulse control, abstract thinking, and learning. The limbic brain is more primitive, more excitatory; the cortex is the 'higher brain,' acting to modulate the limbic brain. Freud's *id* and *ego* reflect our modern understanding of the limbic and cortical brains.

As the years pass, a child's cortex is shaped by her experiences. The activation of and connections between brain cells (neurons) dictate the workings of a child's brain, and experience has a direct effect on which brain cells are activated and how they become linked to one another. Specific environmental cues are required for the proper organization of these connections, and when those cues are missing due to neglect, or come from violent sources, the child's brain ends up disorganized and less functional.

This has been demonstrated time and time again in scientific studies that link brain activity with violent or otherwise antisocial behaviors in children and adults.

Because the brain is a remarkably malleable organ, these kinds of changes—while they may not be reversible—can almost always be compensated for with the right kind of therapy and community support. This will be my focus in the second half of this book.

If a child feels safe and her days are orderly, full of constructive stimulation and loving attention, her cortex develops normally, and over time she becomes more and more able to control her basic impulses. A two-year-old child is likely to hit, bite, or scream when she doesn't get her way, because her cortex hasn't gained its full ability to modulate her impulses. An eight-year-old child's cortical development—in good circumstances—is such that she is able to feel her urge to strike out, but can channel it into more socially acceptable means for getting what she wants. Her ability to think in an abstract manner is well on its way to being established. The older child is also better equipped to handle traumatic experiences, should she end up confronted by one. Good family support from attentive caregivers helps to cushion the blow of traumatic experience, and if this support has been there all along, her brain has been developing the capacity to deal with trauma since her birth.

Violent Trauma: Its Effects on Children

Trauma during childhood shapes the formation of personality, of self-concept, and of the child's vision of the future (or lack thereof). Kardiner, the psychologist who studied shell-shock during and after World War I, described the long-term "diminution of interest and intelligence" caused by "the continuous shrinkage of the field of effective functioning" and the simple joys that can come from being a capable and involved human being. For a child traumatized by violence, the world becomes a dangerous place, and when we are in danger, our worlds shrink. Our energies are directed towards survival and self-protection.

Not altering our function in this way would be like deciding to set up an easel and paint on the deck of a sinking ship. If you don't start thinking about how to get to a lifeboat right quick, you and your artwork—regardless of how brilliant that artwork may be—are going to end up at the bottom of the ocean. Human biology gets this, and it automatically makes drastic changes in the workings of body and mind when danger is afoot.

Dissociation and Development

The younger a child is at the onset of violent trauma, the greater the likelihood that he will respond to that trauma by dissociating. The essence of dissociation is the separation of reality from perception. Very young children talk of "watching" their own abuse, or of putting themselves "in the wall" or in some other place where they do not have to be present for the abuse.

Dissociation is extremely damaging to the developmental process. Coupled with the lack of impulse control that is characteristic of traumatized children, it creates teens and adults with enormous difficulties in the realms of trust, intimacy, self-assertion, and body image. These teens and adults are likely to feel helpless and to see themselves as damaged goods.

Adults who were traumatized as children also tend to lack the ability to feel their feelings. Many have a startling lack of empathy, which some have characterized as "emotional retardation." They have trouble identifying their emotions because they have grown accustomed to ignoring or overriding them to try to control and find safety from violent situations. They may have enormous problems simply caring for their own most fundamental needs—for example, rest and hygiene—while, at the same time, being highly aware of the needs of others. Abuse survivors who are better at protecting themselves do so without the satisfaction that comes from a healthy degree of safety in the world. They protect themselves tenaciously, desperately, as a matter of survival.

Many adult survivors of childhood trauma revisit their traumas again and again, particularly women who were sexually abused and seek out adult relationships with men who abuse them. The younger the person was when the abuse began, the more likely he is to re-enact that abuse throughout his lifetime, either as victim or victimizer. (This is the classic example of the bully who is bullied at home by abusive parents.)

Women who were sexually assaulted or abused as children have been found to be far more likely to be raped or become prostitutes as teens and adults. Their behaviors and choices appear to invite retraumatization. It appears that women who fall into this kind of pattern are attempting to exert control over abusive situations. Unconsciously, she is saying, "If I'm going to be violated, then I'm going to control where, when, and how it happens."

Psychosomatic symptoms often result in the aftermath of violent trauma, and this is especially true of children who are too young to express themselves effectively in the abstract sense—with words. In brain scans of people with post-traumatic stress disorders, exposure to a stimulus that reminds the survivor of their trauma causes increased blood flow to the parts of the brain that are associated with emotion and "fight-or-flight" arousal. At the same time, the utilization of oxygen drops in the region of the cortex responsible for generating words to attach to internal experience. (Rausch et al.) This explains why terrifying events often rob us of the ability to speak. In children who live in an environment bathed in fear, the ability to link feelings to words may be permanently damaged.

During the earliest years of life, children tend towards "magical thinking," where they feel that everything that happens to them is attributable to their own actions or thoughts. Small children who have been abused tend to believe that the abuse was their fault, and that belief may persist for a lifetime. It follows that the abuse survivor will also blame herself for other things that are not her fault, over which she has no control.

Play is a child's way of experimenting with roles and possibilities. Through play, children learn healthy approaches to their own feelings and to situations or issues that are difficult. Children who live bathed in fear lose their ability to play. They have trouble imagining the future. They don't see a world of possibility, but a world where they are helpless, where they have to focus on protecting themselves.

Children who are abused by trusted caregivers lose their foundation for trust. They feel incompetent, worthless, and insignificant. In an attempt to maintain attachment to those caregivers, they may begin to identify with those who abuse them.

The single most important job of a child, from the day it is born, is to engage the love and nurturing of their caregivers. They are wired to do whatever needs to be done in order to hold the attention of those upon whom they are dependent. They will go to great lengths to do so—even if that means perceiving themselves as unlovable, weak, and generally worthy of the abuses they are forced to endure. Intermittent abuse causes a child to identify with her tormentors even more strongly; she is grateful when the abuse doesn't happen, and is thankful to her abuser for not harming her on that occasion.

In traumatized children, the slightest threat triggers fear, arousal, anxiety, and dissociation. Performing well in school when in this condition is practically impossible; children who are hyperaroused often can't sit still in class, and end up being diagnosed with attention deficit/hyperactivity disorder (ADHD). They simply cannot learn in an abstract (cortical) way when their brainstems and autonomic (fight-or-flight) nervous systems are busy trying to keep them safe from harm. I will delve more deeply into the issue of hyperarousal in Chapter Five.

Traumatized children run greater risk of depression, separation anxiety, unremitting grief, ADHD, substance abuse, and phobias compared to children who are not severely traumatized. They are likely to suffer from sleep problems and accompanying daytime deficits in concentration and attentiveness. Social withdrawal, accompanied by intense longing for intimacy, is common in trauma victims of all ages. And, most importantly for the purposes of this book, children who have been violated or witnessed violence are more likely to turn violent themselves.

Violence Breeds Violence

According to Bruce Perry, a leading theorist in the field of trauma therapy, "modern history is characterized by increasingly efficient, systematic and institutionalized violence." (Perry BD, "Incubated in Terror: Neurodevelopmental Factors in the Cycle of Violence," *Children, Youth, and Violence: the Search for Solutions,* J. Osofsky, Ed., Guilford Press, New York NY:124-28, 1997.) The institutionalized violence of the Holocaust, where millions of Jews and other so-called "inferior" people were killed systematically (often after being worked nearly to death for the profit of their captors) in Nazi death camps, was unlike anything seen before it. African-American slavery can also be considered institutional violence, and the systems that kept it in place for nearly two centuries were nothing if not efficient and institutionalized.

Where at one time, wars were fought by brutal hand-to-hand combat, today we can wipe out an entire nation with bombs fired from hundreds of miles away. A single assailant with an automatic weapon can kill a dozen people in the blink of an eye. Terrorists hijacked three commercial airplanes and killed more than 3,000 people on a single day of breathtaking violence—September 11, 2001. It's a frightening world, and children know this. They live in an atmosphere of fear and distrust unlike any that has existed before.

On a smaller scale, domestic and acquaintance violence still happens the old-fashioned way: face-to-face, hand-to-hand, and often in the presence of or against children. Abuse, neglect, and exposure to domestic violence are far bigger social problems than community violence (such as gang warfare) and predatory violence (such as sniper attacks or carjackings), but the latter two problems get a lot more press.

Perhaps—and here, I'll take a hint from Freud's recantation of his early theory that hysteria was caused by childhood sexual abuse—we are afraid as a culture to take an honest look at how children are being treated. Perhaps our culture is not ready to face the vast scale on which children are neglected, exposed to family violence, or otherwise hurt by those who are meant to care for and nurture them. Until we are willing to do so, however, the problem will continue to get worse, because *those who do the community and predatory violence are almost invariably the ones who were subjected to domestic violence and neglect as children.* (Perry, ibid.)

Virtually every criminal I have interviewed in prisons—and there have been hundreds—has a history of domestic or community violence. When a child is bathed in violence, he does not learn how to manage the problems that always arise in the context of relationships. He has seen conflict handled in one way: through the use of physical force. Bessel van der Kolk:

When the inevitable disagreements and power struggles that are part of any relationship cannot be managed with either total control or perfect submission, people with abuse histories tend to be unable to articulate their wishes, to fail to understand the other person's point of view, and to be unable to compromise. Having had little experience with nonviolent resolution of differences, partners in such relationships often alternate between an expecta-

tion of perfect behavior leading to perfect harmony, and a state of helplessness in which all verbal communication seems futile.

—Van der Kolk BA, McFarlane AC, and Weisaeth L, *Traumatic Stress: The Effects of Overwhelming Experience on Mind, Body, and Society,* Guilford Press, London/New York: 1996.

An abuse survivor (or a child who is threatened by community violence on a regular basis) might handle this helplessness by retreating, but he also might turn to violence. This is far more likely in children who have also suffered some amount of neglect. *The very adaptations that a child must make in order to survive an existence in a violent household or a violent neighborhood increase that child's chances of becoming violent himself.* He becomes hypervigilant and loses his capacity to feel his feelings. He loses the ability to control his impulsive desires to strike out—which all of us have time and again—because his cerebral cortex is underdeveloped. He's constantly on the lookout for danger, and often finds it.

In the case of abuse by caregivers or parents, the child's dissociation enables him to continue to suffer the abuse while still remaining under their care. The child doesn't know there is any other way. Heartbreakingly, abused children love their parents and are strongly attached to them, and often resist being removed from the homes where they have been so badly treated. They know nothing else. This is their model of family life.

A child who can't control his impulses because of a poorly developed cortex might strike out at another child for what seems to all observers like no big deal—an insult, eye contact held for a moment too long, or a slight that would roll off of another child's back. Another child might insist that his violent behavior was necessary to protect himself against aggression from someone else.

Some children who engage in bullying or attacks on other children report being soothed or calmed by doing so; experimental evidence shows that hyperaroused boys from traumatic backgrounds show a decrease in heart rate when they become aggressive. Girls, on the other hand, appear to be soothed by self-destructive behaviors such as cutting. Research has shown that in hyperaroused children, heart rate is consistently higher than normal, and that violent "acting out" in boys and self-destructive behavior in girls actually causes the heart rate to drop. It has also been found that girls' heart rates drop when they are allowed to tell a therapist about the traumas they've suffered, while the boys' heart rates went up. Telling their stories made the boys feel more vulnerable to danger.

Conclusions

Have we answered the question of why children turn violent? For the most part, we have. But there is another part of the equation to consider. Being violated or being traumatized by exposure to violence makes a child violent, but there are cultural factors in play here as well. A child who is hypervigilant, dissociated, and impulsive because of abuse, neglect, or other traumatic experience is more likely to engage in defensive, impulsive, or predatory violence, and these types of violence are facilitated by the beliefs of the person who turns violent. According to Bruce Perry, these beliefs include "racism, sexism, misogyny, children as property, idealization of violent heroes, cultural tolerance or child maltreatment, tribalism, jingoism, nationalism." (Perry, ibid.)

Beliefs are taught, handed down through generations just as trauma is passed along from parent to child. If we are to help today's traumatized children to break the chain of trauma that began generations ago, we must not only address the trauma itself, but the belief systems that create targets for violence.

This Is Your Brain After Traumatic Stress

Studies of people with PTSD have found changes in the activity and even in the size of certain parts of the brain.

Decreased hippocampal volume:
Activation of the amygdala during flashbacks:
Right-hemispheric lateralization:

Also add: fearful child puts forth a defiant stance—may be seen as willful, controlling; adult responds by becoming more angry and demanding; child may move into 'mini-psychotic' state from non-verbal signals he is getting

Chapter Five

Fight, Flee, Dissociate, Somatize
The Consequences of Trauma

The organ which allows the child victim to adapt to any violent trauma is the brain—just as the brain is the origin for the violent behaviors of the victimizer. How is it that the very neurobiological adaptations which allow the child to survive violence may, as the child grows older, result in an increased tendency to be violent? It is not the finger pulling the trigger that kills; it is not the penis that rapes—it is the brain. In order to understand violence, we need to understand the organization and functioning of its birthplace—the brain.

—Bruce Perry, "Incubated in Terror: Neurodevelopmental Factors in the 'Cycle of Violence,'" In: Children, Youth and Violence: The Search For Solutions, *J. Osofsky, Ed., Guilford Press, New York, pp. 124-148:1997.*

As we have seen from previous chapters, the experiences of children have powerful effects on their development and behaviors. Some argue that brain development is affected by environmental factors even prenatally—in fact, a field of study called *prenatal and perinatal psychology* has begun to study the influence of events before, during, and following birth. Whether or not putting headphones playing Mozart over an expectant mother's belly has any significant impact on a child's future intelligence, there is absolutely no debate over the impact of experiences in childhood and infancy on the development of mental and emotional faculties in children.

A single traumatic event can change the whole course of a child's life. One man I interviewed—one who was in prison for murder—told me about having been abandoned as an infant for two days. Although I knew that he could not possibly have any conscious recollection of an event that occurred when he was only a few months old, he described it as though he could, and tears welled up in his eyes as he told his story. He intuitively knew that this experience had been enough to destroy him.

The life-changing impact of trauma having been established, science is still exploring the ways in which traumatic experiences actually affect the physiological development of the brain, and how they alter the activity of neurotransmitters and hormones. Little doubt exists that trauma leaves lasting marks on these variables—marks that go deeper and last longer in some people than in others. As we move towards an understanding of exactly how this comes about, we move towards an answer to the questions: are these changes permanent? If not, can this kind of irreversible damage be overcome?

Yes, some of these changes may well be permanent; but fortunately, yes, it seems that most can be overcome.

The brain and body are both remarkably malleable, and they yearn for a life that is comfortable, balanced, loving, and happy. But if the impact of traumatic events aren't dealt with promptly—if a traumatized child is not treated and cared for properly while still a child—the probability of complete healing is not great. The more time passes between trauma and intervention, the greater its hold on the person, and the more difficult it becomes to reverse its effects.

It has been said that a brief window exists for trauma intervention that will enable the traumatized person to make a complete recovery. If proper counseling and support are delivered within 48 hours of the trauma, it seems that the lasting physiological effects that create vulnerability to PTSD can be bypassed. As you might guess, this rarely happens for disenfranchised, impoverished children who live with the threat of (and reality of) family and community violence, day in and day out.

In this chapter, I will share what is known about the effect of persistent trauma and stress on the physical body, in the context of two of the most common symptoms of PTSD: hyperarousal and dissociation. I will describe the impact these symptoms have on emotional development and intelligence. Somatization, a rarer symptom, will also be addressed.

Mind, brain, and body are all of one piece; none can be left out of any discussion on trauma, and anyone who makes divisions between these pieces of human beings is doing so to make an academic or scientific point, not to deal with the real world.

Definitions

Let's clearly define the terms we will be using in this chapter: *hyperarousal, dissociation,* and *somatization.* I have addressed all three of these terms briefly in earlier chapters, but let's review them here:

Hyperarousal is also known as *hypervigilance.* A hyperaroused person is always looking out for danger and quick to react when any danger is sensed—often, perceiving real danger where none exists. In this state, something as benign as direct eye contact, a hand on the shoulder, or a criticism are blown far out of proportion, and the person reacts accordingly.

The hypervigilant person is in constant "fight-or-flight" mode. In many ways, that person has regressed to a more primitive, animalistic state, where he perceives physical cues rather than more complex, abstract verbal cues. His cortical brain takes a backseat to his limbic brain.

Both children and adults can become hypervigilant in response to trauma. Children who are prematurely separated from their primary caregiver—usually the mother—are at increased risk of becoming hypervigilant. This makes perfect sense, as a child who is not protected by his mother is going to have to take on the responsibility of self-protection before it's developmentally appropriate that he does so.

Chronically hyperaroused people lose the ability to interpret their own emotions. The basic function of feelings is to get people to pay attention to their environment so that they can take adaptive action. For example: Raheem is feeling romantic love towards Lisa, which tells him to do all he can to make her his romantic partner. Lisa, on the other hand, might feel revulsion because Raheem prefers not to bathe, and this drives her to take her own adaptive action: removing herself as far from Raheem as she possibly can.

Emotional arousal is part of Nature's design, a reaction to the environment that is designed to stimulate goal-directed action. Instead of seeing the signal of arousal as a sign that it's time to use the cortical brain to figure out how to adapt, the traumatized person jumps directly into fight, flight, or freeze mode. The constant "jacking up" of hyperarousal reduces the person's ability to recognize other emotional signals. Healthy relationship, under these circumstances, becomes difficult or impossible. So does performing well in school or at a demanding job, or being a good parent.

It is not unusual for hypervigilant individuals to resort to avoidance behaviors, effectively shrinking the scope of their lives down to avoid things that remind them of their trauma.

In many ways, *dissociation* is the flip-side of hypervigilance. An individual with PTSD usually flips back and forth from numb, dissociated unresponsiveness to intermittent hyperarousal and back again. Traumatized people tend to incorporate both dissociation and hyperarousal into their responses; generally, females tend more towards the dissociative, anxious, and unhappy, while males tend more towards hyperarousal and aggression.

Dissociation is a split that occurs between the self that observes the world and the self that experiences it. It often occurs in the moment of traumatic experience, when the pain of what is happening become so unbearable that the person being traumatized steps out of the experience and observes it from outside herself.

Three subcategories of dissociation have been defined:

Primary dissociation describes the split between sensory and emotional aspects of trauma that can occur during the traumatic event. Instead of perceiving the event as a whole, it is perceived as fragments of sensory information: sights, odors, sounds, sensations. Afterwards, the survivor suffers from equally fragmented memories—intrusive recollections, flashbacks, and nightmares.

Secondary dissociation describes a separation between the self that observes and the self that experiences. This is what is being described when trauma survivors talk of "leaving their bodies" or otherwise protecting themselves from pain by observing their traumas as spectators rather than as victims.

As time goes by, the breadth of that separation increases and becomes incorporated into the trauma survivor's personality. A split remains, so that some aspects of that person's personality incorporate the pain and fear of their traumatic experience, while others seem unaware of it.This is *tertiary dissociation.*

When a trauma victim dissociates during the event itself, her chances of developing post-traumatic stress disorder are greater. Dissociation serves the purpose of numbing the impact of the trauma, at the expense of being able to integrate it into one's overall experience. This kind of integration is the only thing that will heal the wounds that trauma leaves behind.

Dissociative adaptations include a broad range of responses to traumatic experience. Any mental mechanism that disengages a person from what is happening in the external world and tunes him into his internal world is considered a dissociative mechanism: daydreaming, fantasy, 'watching from outside the body,' going to a 'different place,' or 'watching a movie' of one's experience are all forms of dissociation.

In extreme states of dissociation, a person may faint, become catatonic (frozen) or may enter what is known as a *fugue state.* Fugue is defined as an episode of altered consciousness that causes the individual to wander; he may do so for hours or days, and does not remember it afterwards.

Multiple personality disorder—an extreme form of dissociation—is rare. The person suffering from multiple personality disorder was subjected to childhood abuse so extreme that her personality emerged in a completely fragmented way. The child who becomes an MPD sufferer becomes so adept at dissociating that she develops two or more distinct personalities. Within the individual patient, some of the personalities are more aggressive and defensive, with others that are more passive and yielding. A milder form of this disorder is known as *borderline personality disorder,* where moods, actions, beliefs, and thoughts are unstable and often conflicting. In BPD, the disparate characteristics develop within the same personality.

A person who is used to dissociating may find that his pain is numbed, but that he is also cut off from happier feelings. Dissociated people report feeling numb, dead, or "on auto-pilot."

They may commit violent acts against others or themselves just to *feel* something.

Dissociation is as Dangerous as Hypervigilance

Dissociation is not as great a social problem as hyperarousal. Neither is a phenomenon known as *learned helplessness,* where an abused person gives up trying to control his world and sinks into a state of defeat. Those who dissociate or give up on life completely aren't so likely to commit violence. They are, however, at greater risk of being completely defeated by trauma. Trauma survivors who become hypervigilant and tend to lash out or otherwise seek attention are at least trying to remain engaged, trying to get some control, some foothold in a world that has not made a safe space for them.

This being the case, why focus attention on healing those who are dissociated? Why not deal with violence by targeting those who are primarily hyperaroused? Because dissociation is dangerous in that it separates feelings from actions. A dissociated parent may not be likely to lash out in violence, but she very well may end up detached from and neglectful of her children. She may end up in an abusive relationship and fail to protect her children from the violence that comes of it. A dissociated person has trouble being a contributing member of the clan.

Remember that we are dealing with trauma at a cultural level here. In order to stop the cycle of violence in the African-American community, we must address trauma in every manifestation. We must help not only those who may do violence because of having been violated, but also those who have given up on life and are willing to step aside as others do violence. We need the help of each set of hands, each heart and mind in the clan, and this means bringing dissociated people back to the land of the living.

Somatization is the body's way of communicating to the brain that a traumatic event needs to be dealt with, that healing is necessary. Unexplained physical symptoms such as vomiting, abdominal pain, nausea, bloating, diarrhea, pain (headache, musculoskeletal, or with intercourse), shortness of breath, heart palpitations, dizziness, difficulty swallowing, vision changes, paralysis, muscle weakness, lack of sexual desire, impotence, and menstrual problems can all be the result of unresolved traumatic stress. Most of Freud and Janet's hysterics had somatization symptoms. This particular aspect of PTSD is proof positive that mental states can have extremely powerful effects on the workings of the physical body.

Most of the trauma survivors who report these kinds of symptoms are females, and symptoms usually begin before the age of 30. They are plagued for years with symptoms that can't be medically explained. They are frustrated by physicians who repeatedly tell them, "There is nothing wrong with you," when they know perfectly well that there *is* something wrong. Eventually, they begin to lose faith in their bodies' signals. They are labeled hypochondriacs or fakers, but the truth is that an expanding realm of scientific research—*psychoneuroimmunology*—is showing how incredibly potent the effects of the mind can be on the immune system, the nervous system, and the digestive system. Being chronically stressed can and does directly cause physical illness.

It's Not "All In Their Heads"

Humans are unique among animals. We have undergone a tremendous amount of social evolution since our prehistoric ancestors evolved. We pass along an enormous amount of sociocultural information to our offspring—information that has little to do with the hard-wiring of our genes and everything to do with the mores and expectations of individual cultures.

The environment in which a child is raised has everything to do with what that child becomes. Recent attempts to find genetic "markers" for everything from aggression to alcoholism to anxiety to depression to obesity may eventually yield some fruit, but any genetic theories about most diseases tend to fall far short of explaining the disease's existence or pattern of influence. For example: much is made of the link between breast cancer and genetics, but the truth is that only a small fraction of people who end up being diagnosed with breast cancer have any sort of genetic predisposition. A great many environmental factors are at play, and those factors are just beginning to be understood.

It's especially easy to look at differences in disease rates between races and attribute those differences to genetics. The first, most glaring problem with this is that the genetic differences between races are miniscule. The genetic differences between humans and *apes* are miniscule!

They simply aren't enough to explain why African-Americans tend towards more problems with obesity, heart disease, diabetes, and high blood pressure. (More on this topic in Chapter Seven.)

The most likely truth about genes and disease is that certain genetic factors may make a person slightly more vulnerable to a particular condition, but that the environment—the events and situations and settings and relationships a person encounters in his life—dictates whether that vulnerability is ever exploited.

This having been said, let's look at the ways in which environment can alter the physical body. We know that psychological trauma has far-reaching effects, but do these effects have a basis in actual physiological changes?

This question has been a subject of debate in psychology for a long time. During recent years, government has launched public awareness campaigns designed to "de-stigmatize" mental illness, to describe it as something that is the result of a physical imbalance or flaw in biochemistry, not something that is "all in your head." Let's recognize that, knowing what we know today, there is no such thing as "all in your head." The body and mind are always linked. If something is out of kilter in the mind, there are causes and effects that involve the body.

The natural outgrowth of this movement has been an almost exclusive focus on the use of psychoactive drugs for the treatment of psychological problems. Antidepressants and anti-anxiety drugs are being used by an unprecedented number of adults and increasingly younger children.Teens and children are estimated to make up five percent of those who use the most popular antidepressants—the selective serotonin uptake inhibitors, or SSRIs, such as Prozac, Zoloft, Paxil, and Celexa.

While drugs can help in the short-term, and while in rare cases they are absolutely necessary for the long-term, they aren't the answer to the PTSD problem, or to most of the more common psychological complaints (anxiety, depression, attention deficit disorder). They may help people to feel better, but they don't help them heal. PTSD, anxiety, depression, and ADHD can all be healed.

As we learned in Chapter Four, lack of appropriate nurturing in infancy and childhood has direct effects on the development of the cortex, increasing the likelihood that it will be unable to modulate arousal. But what about traumatic experience? When a young girl is forced to have sex with her father, does this actually change her neurochemistry? When a young boy watches a friend get shot, does his body change as well as his mind?

Unequivocally, yes. Research is demonstrating that dissociation and hyperarousal are distinctly physical processes that arise from changes in the activity of neurotransmitters and hormones. Developing brains become developed brains by interacting with cues from the external environment. Neurotransmitters and hormones are made in response to these cues, and in response to their interactions within the body.

Neurotransmitters are chemicals made in the cells of the nervous system. Their job is to move information from nerve cell to nerve cell. Serotonin and dopamine are the primary neurotransmitters we will talk about in this chapter.

Hormones are chemicals made in glands that influence the workings of tissues throughout the body. Hormones are carried through the bloodstream and latch onto receptors, which are like a lock that fits the hormone "key." When that key fits into that lock, changes are initiated in the tissues where the receptor is.

As a result of these complex processes, neurons (brain and nerve cells) divide, move around within the brain, form connections, and take on various responsibilities in the brain. This process transforms the largely undifferentiated, unorganized nervous system with which we are all born into a mature, functioning adult nervous system. Traumatic experience disrupts this process.

Catecholamines and Cortisol

Hypervigilance involves very specific physiological changes. Heart rate and body temperature rise and muscle tone increases. The hyperaroused person is quick to startle and has trouble sleeping. In one study, children who had experienced trauma had a resting heart rate of 104 (normal is 90 or lower). In boys, heart rate rose to an average of 122 beats per minute during a non-intrusive interview about their trauma. In girls, heart rate started out at 98 BPM and fell to 84 BPM during the interview. (Perry et al, in press)

In a study of boys who lived in a residential center following prolonged, extreme exposure to domestic violence, researchers asked the boys about specific violent events they had been involved in (as perpetrators). The boys' descriptions of their feelings during these events brought the researchers to the conclusion that taking violent action had a soothing, calming effect on them. They became dissociated, detached from their pain. Dissociation can be blissful in the face of the anxious fearfulness of hyperarousal—this is why so many people with PTSD turn to alcohol or drugs, which reliably produce states of dissociation and calm.

Another research group followed a group of traumatized children from age 15 through 29. They found that those who ended up committing criminal acts had lower heart rates than those who did not. It was as if, by "taking control" through acts of violence, these traumatized people were able to feel themselves to be in control, perhaps for the very first time. (Raine et al, 1995)

These physical manifestations of hyperarousal come about because of changes in *catecholamines* and *cortisol.* Catecholamines are chemicals made in the adrenal glands, located just above the kidneys. They spur a "fight or flight" physical response, quickly raising blood pressure, breathing rate, and heart rate, and causing the pupils to dilate and the brain to be more alert. They decrease blood flow to the digestive organs and skin, while increasing blood flow to muscles, lungs, and brain, as well as stimulating the breakdown of stored fat and carbohydrate for use as fuel. In people with PTSD, simple reminders of the trauma elicit extreme versions of the catecholamine response.

The catecholamine response is only designed for short-term arousal—enough time to get out of danger. If catecholamine release is continually high because of post-traumatic stress, the body eventually begins to compensate by decreasing the number of binding sites for these chemicals. They fail to have the same effects. It is as though the body understands that it has to change its balance point to avoid being burned out.

Cortisol is a hormone that modulates the body's response to environmental stresses. Animals who have had their adrenal glands removed can die from the effects of sudden stress, and humans who have taken large doses of synthetic cortisol-like drugs to treat asthma, autoimmune diseases, or cancer can die if they stop abruptly (the drugs cause the body's natural cortisol production to fall dramatically). Like the catecholamines, cortisol is produced by the adrenal glands during periods of stress; greater stress elicits greater cortisol production. Cortisol's short-term effects are not well understood—it may simply act to potentiate the effects of catecholamines—but its role in mediating the body's response to long-term, chronic stress is much better understood.

Let's imagine a man stranded on a lifeboat, out in the ocean, starving, sunburnt, exhausted, anxious, and despairing. His adrenal glands become slightly swollen and pump out extra cortisol. The cortisol ensures that his brain and heart continue to receive the fuel they need by making glucose (sugars), the brain's preferred fuel, out of amino acids (components of protein). Muscle tissue and connective tissue (such as bone) are broken down to provide amino acids for this purpose.

Now, let's imagine the man after he's been rescued. The trauma of his ordeal stays with him. He no longer feels safe in the world. His cortisol levels are around normal when he is not facing stress, but they rise more dramatically when he is stressed. The number of cortisol receptors on the cells throughout his body decreases, just as catecholamine receptors do, but the number of cortisol receptors in the hippocampus increase. It seems that in people with PTSD, the cortisol system increases its overall sensitivity, and this increase in sensitivity allows space for it to relax between stressful times.

It has been proposed that cortisol actually works as a sort of "anti-stress" hormone that shuts off other biological responses to stress. Low levels of cortisol during stressful times leads to a relative overload of catecholamines, which in turn sends the person into fight-or-flight mode.

A large body of research has established a connection between chronic stimulation of cortisol and catecholamines and chronic disease. In children, obesity, depression, and permanent damage to the hippocampal region of the brain have been linked to oversecretion of these hormones. Adults with high cortisol are more likely to be hypertensive, diabetic, and to develop Alzheimer's disease or coronary artery disease.

The body is always striving for balance. When a person's environment is changed by traumatic stress, certain physiological reactions take place: catecholamine and cortisol levels rise, along with heart rate, blood pressure, muscle tone, and respiratory rate. When these changes persist for some time—when the stress stays with the trauma survivor because of PTSD or recurrence of the trauma—these physiological changes become the norm. States become traits. The body adjusts, adapting to this new level of functioning.

There are two kinds of balance. There's the tightrope walker gliding confidently along under the big top with a net below to catch her. Then there's the daredevil who walks on a rope strung across a windswept 500-foot gully, balancing a stack of plates on each end of the stick she holds for balance, wearing a blindfold.

The person who is dealing with traumatic stress may achieve some new kind of balance, but it is rarely a healthful one. It is achieved through avoidance of significant activities and relationships, through shutting down connections between emotions and actions, and physical changes that keep the traumatized person hypervigilant or dissociated.

Neurotransmitters and Post-Traumatic Stress

Girls who suffer from traumatic stress are more likely than boys to engage in a practice known as self-cutting. They report feeling empty and numb—in psychological terminology, dissociated—and they say that cutting themselves affords them relief from their numbness.

Bessel van der Kolk and co-workers did a fascinating experiment involving eight girls who engaged in self-cutting. The researchers evaluated the pain sensitivity of the girls when they were having very strong urges to cut themselves, and found that no stimulus (within ethical limits) caused the girls to report any significant sensation of pain.

Opiates: substances that numb pain responses and bring about feelings of calm.

Endogenous opiates: opiates that are made within the body, such as endorphins.

Exogenous opiates: opiates that are substances foreign to the body that have opiate effects when taken in; for example, alcohol, cocaine, heroin, and marijuana.

They then administered a drug called naltrexone, which interferes with the activity of endogenous opiates. The girls were then able to feel pain. This study provides good evidence that endogenous opiates are responsible for dissociation. Dissociation can be predictably produced with drugs and alcohol—another piece of evidence that indicates a biological basis for this mental shift.

Dopamine: A neurotransmitter that mediates the dissociative response.

Serotonin: A neurotransmitter that mediates mood and other variables; believed to be low in depressed individuals. Traumatized animals demonstrate decreased serotonin activity. Serotonin levels are increased by the most popular class of antidepressants, the selective serotonin reuptake inhibitors–including Prozac, Zoloft, Celexa, and others.

Sympathetic nervous system: the aspect of the nervous system that is activated during fight-or-flight (or freeze) responses.

Parasympathetic nervous system: the balancing aspect of the nervous system that counteracts sympathetic activity, lowering heart rate and blood pressure and having a calming effect.

Vagal tone: the level at which the parasympathetic nervous system is activated. Vagal tone varies from person to person, and can be increased with exercise and meditation.

The threshold for dissociation varies from person to person. One might dissociate at the slightest trauma, while another might resist dissociation unless the trauma is completely terrifying. It is believed that a neurotransmitter called *dopamine* interacts with activity of the brainstem (the most primitive part of the brain that orchestrates basic bodily functions) to create a dissociative state. During the trauma, cortisol and catecholamines rise just as they do to create a hyperaroused state, but the parasympathetic nervous system is activated. Vagal tone increases dramatically—sometimes so dramatically that fainting results. At the same time, endogenous opiates are produced, deadening sensations of pain.

States Become Traits

Any psychological state that hangs around long enough will become integrated into personality. When you look at the changes in neurotransmitter and central nervous system activity that occur with dissociative and hyperaroused states, this makes perfect sense. These systems become locked into a dissociative or hyperaroused pattern. The earlier in life the trauma is initiated, the more firmly locked-in this pattern becomes.

The body strives to find its balance, no matter where that balance point may be. This is what makes traumatic stress so hard to treat: in order to reestablish a healthier balance, we must first find a way to disrupt the unhealthy balance that has been established, both psychologically and biologically. And trauma survivors hang tenuously on to the balance they have struggled to reach. Any attempts to upset it feel like attacks and further violations to these people.

The Problem of Addiction

Traumatized people often turn to alcohol and other drugs, especially those who feel hyperaroused by their trauma. In a study by the National Center for Chronic Disease Prevention and Health Promotion, it was found that each incidence of adverse childhood experience doubled to quadrupled the likelihood that drug use would be initiated.

African-Americans are no more likely to initiate drug use than people of other races, despite the historical and current traumas they suffer as a race. In fact, they are *less* likely to use illicit drugs or to binge-drink than whites. According to data from the CDC, white high school students are:

7 times more likely than blacks to have used cocaine;
8 times more likely than blacks to have used crack;
10 times more likely than blacks to have used heroin;
twice as likely as blacks to binge-drink;
and nearly twice as likely as blacks to drive drunk.

Race divisions aside, the famous slogan "Just Say No" takes on a hint of ridiculousness in the face of trauma. For someone who has survived abuse, neglect, or other forms of traumatic experience, the pain they are feeling is simply too much to bear, and as soon as they realize that drugs and alcohol can take away that pain, is it any wonder that they turn to them?

The politicians who create anti-drug programs in this country have a lot to learn about the roots of addiction. When white men from privileged backgrounds begin to make moral judgements upon the rest of us, it is all too easy to question their ability to comprehend that which they presume to judge. "Just say no?" How about, "Let's get real?"

Depression, Anxiety, Self-Destructive Behaviors, and Trauma

Depression and anxiety disorders are being diagnosed and treated (with drugs, mostly) in unprecedented numbers of people today. It seems that every time I turn around, a new depressive or anxiety disorder is being defined in the psychology lexicon. What is the relationship between trauma, depression, anxiety, and self-destructive behaviors?

In the words of researchers from the Emory University school of Medicine, "early life traumatic events, occurring during a period of neuronal plasticity, appear to permanently render neuroendocrine stress response systems supersensitive." This increases the long-term risk of additional psychological problems, including depression, anxiety, self-cutting, eating disorders, and psychotic (violent) tendencies.

David R. Williams has written a detailed review of the interactions between socioeconomic status, race, and family in African-Americans. He examines the prevalence of psychiatric disorders in various races, based on studies involving almost 20,000 adults interviewed in five mental health catchment areas in the U.S. The studies

> *found little variation in rates of disorder by race. Rates of depressive disorders, alcohol and drug abuse are very similar for blacks and whites, with a tendency for some white rates to be higher...The overall evidence on black mental health is somewhat surprising. African Americans are disproportionately exposed to social conditions considered to be important risk factors for physical and mental illness...At the same time, blacks do not have higher rates of suicide or higher rates of mental illness than whites. And among the poor, white males have higher rates of mental illness than black males.*
>
> —David R. Williams, "African-American Mental Health: Persisting Questions and Paradoxical Findings"

Other research suggests a rising incidence of suicide among African-Americans. Young African-American women are less likely to cut themselves or suffer from eating disorders than young white women, but they appear to be more vulnerable to self-destructive sexual promiscuity than white girls. They are more likely to become unwed teen mothers than white girls, as well.

Let's just presume for a moment that African-Americans are, indeed, at lower risk of certain psychological diagnoses, as some of the research suggests.

What are the implications of this? In my opinion, this bodes well for the future of African-Americans. We made good slaves because of our strength, spirit, and resilience, and today, we still have these characteristics to fall back on, to lift us up when things are difficult. With the right support from one another, from the community at large, and from the psychology community, there is no reason to believe that we cannot overcome the burden of traumatic experience.

Chapter Six

The Science of Mother (and Father) Love

Everyone has an opinion about how best to raise babies up to be children and children up to be adults. Every mother has been given more than her fair share of unsolicited parenting advice, and more likely than not, she ends up doling the same kind of advice to those who are just embarking on the parenting journey. Such advice usually falls into one of two categories: things I did that worked, and things I wish I had done differently.

Parenting styles change from generation to generation, but it's virtually impossible for the apple to fall too far from the tree. Our most basic instincts about parenting arise from the way in which we ourselves have been parented. In the years when our brains are most malleable, long before we find ourselves leafing through those parenting books at the bookstore, we store away most of the information that we will eventually use to parent our own children.

Parenting isn't something that is best learned from a book. Being a good parent requires both the experience of having been parented and the experience of having children yourself. It's a process of trial and error, and sometimes—even under the best of circumstances—raising children is difficult. It can feel like wandering through a dark maze full of dead-ends. If our own experiences as children were traumatic because of the way we were parented, however, we may need to start from square one, learning parenting from books like this one, or from parenting classes.

This is particularly true of parents who are stuck in less than optimal circumstances—poverty, an environment full of violence and fear, the absence of a father, or not having been parented appropriately. For those parents who suffered abuse or witnessed violence as children, parenting well presents unique challenges.

The African-American community needs help parenting its children. I hope that by this point, I have been able to establish that this community has been disproportionately harmed by traumas that began with slavery. Today's African-American parenting styles continue to reflect this intergenerational trauma, and *culturally relevant* solutions are desperately needed. Typically, government-run parenting education classes don't take into account the African-American cultural characteristics that are a source of pride and pleasure to so many people. If parenting differently means giving up our blackness, many will be unwilling to do what is necessary.

Breaking the cycle of intergenerational trauma is only possible if today's African-American parents give their children the tools they need to avoid traumatic situations whenever possible; and, if such situations are unavoidable, to build the strength of their minds, hearts, and souls to deal with traumas past, present, and future.

Carl Bell on Resiliency

In his writings and lectures, Dr. Carl Bell emphasizes the importance of teaching children to be resilient in the face of whatever life brings them. Dr. Bell describes resiliency in terms of the following characteristics:

a having curiosity and intellectual mastery;
b having compassion—with detachment;
c having the ability to conceptualize;
d obtaining the conviction of one's right to survive;
e possessing the ability to remember and invoke images of good and sustaining figures;
f having the ability to be in touch with affects [feelings], not denying or suppressing major affects as they arise;
g having a goal to live for;
h having the ability to attract and use support;
i possessing a vision of the possibility of restoration of civilized moral order;

- **j** having the need and ability to help others;
- **k** having an affective repertory [a wide range of emotions];
- **l** being resourceful;
- **m** being altruistic towards others; and
- **n** having the capacity to turn traumatic helplessness into learned helpfulness.

These characteristics will blossom in the child who is parented well: the child who is firmly guided without being controlled; the child who is taught to be disciplined without being neurotic; the child who knows that his parent(s) and community members are there for him, rooting for him, and willing to help him grow into a stable and successful adult.

The Dichotomy of African-American Parenting

Does any of this sound familiar to you?

"Do what I say…and do it NOW."
"Because I said so."
"Don't give me no backtalk!"
"Quit your crying, now."
"Any more sass from you, and I'll give you a whipping!"

African-American parenting is, traditionally, authoritarian. Children are expected to do as they are told, when they are told. If they try to speak up for themselves, they end up in even more trouble for talking back. They may be scolded for crying or being afraid.

On the other hand, many modern African-American parents—including those who are authoritarian—coddle their children, especially their male children. They overprotect them. Male children are often treated like royalty by overworked parents, particularly if they are being raised by a single mother. These overindulged male children grow up thinking of themselves as kings, without having had any real king's training.

They find themselves ill-prepared to deal with relationships. To the world they display a bravado that gets them in trouble with their communities and with the law, and they don't have the ability to maintain good relationships outside the home. Many black men I have interviewed in prison have a deep loathing for their mothers. They know that their own mothers' overprotectiveness has a lot to do with their own failures in life and in relationships.

Both the authoritarianism and the coddling can be traced back to slave days. Slave children had to be taught to obey without question, because they were expected to do so with their masters and mistresses. Boys were often separated from their mothers during slavery. Today's African-American mothers still feel the deep fear of their male children being taken from them by some power beyond their control. They cling tightly, but in the process, they fail to prepare their sons to be men: to become heads of household, to protect and provide by mainstream America's definition.

Crime, violence, and incarceration are definitely partly attributable to rampant trauma in the African-American community, but they also spring from this place: boys who cannot control their impulses go out into the world, looking like men, having sex like men, but they feel entitled to have whatever they want, when they want it—because their mothers pampered them too much.

Mothers Cannot Teach Boys to Be Men

A big part of the problem is that more than half of African-American children are parented by single mothers. Mothers are, by their nature, coddling and protective. This is our role in the duality of parenting. The father's role is to transform boys into men. *African-American women cannot take their sons into manhood.* Our Creator did not design us to do that! We are not equipped to cross our boys over into their rites of passage.

Whether we like it or not, children take on the behaviors and the persona of their gender. If you hand a baby doll to a boy and to a girl, the boy is more likely to play catch with it than change its diaper. If you hand a toy gun to a boy and to a girl, they will play with them in very different ways—regardless of what they have been taught by their parents. This has been the reality in the childrearing lives of many a frustrated parent who wanted to raise their children unlimited by "gender constraints." If we can see these so-called "constraints" as sources of power, we will be better equipped to raise healthy, happy men and women from our boys and girls.

Male and female humans are wired differently, and thank goodness for that. Both have unique strengths that are needed in the world. Girls are wired to nurture and take care of others, and boys are wired to protect and provide. There's no harm in this duality, although the women's equality movement has asked us to believe that a woman and a man can do all of the same things in life, equally well. Many of the problems modern families are dealing with can be traced back to this mistaken notion.

African-American boys raised by single mothers see themselves as heads of household long before they are ready to hold this position, and they hold it without having been taught by their own fathers how to do so. They take the king's throne too quickly, without having been trained by the king they would replace. These boys are also forced to take on the pain that the father would have to shoulder if he were doing his job—the pain of conducting an adult, married life, often under stressful circumstances.

It follows that African-American boys must have strong male influence in their lives. If parents are separated and Dad is around and willing, boy children should be raised under his roof, with visitation from the mother, starting at around the age of 10. If there is another woman in Dad's life, the child's mother needs to be strong in maintaining her own unique place in the boy's life.

Remember the film "Boyz in the Hood?" The single black mother took her ten-year-old son to live with his father, recognizing that she could not give him what he needed. The adjustment was difficult; the son was used to being coddled, and the father was masculine and rigid, but the boy needed exactly that environment to grow into a man.

Of course, there may be the small issue of the child's father never having been crossed over into manhood himself. He may never have been taught how to treat women, or how to be strong. If this is the case, the father is ill-equipped to teach his own sons.

If Dad is absent or inadequate to bring sons into manhood, single mothers still have some options. They can get their boys into military school. They can get their boys involved in all-male activities such as school sports. The key is to remove the boy from weak influences as often as possible.

I'm probably going to take a lot of heat for referring to African-American women as "weak," but let's face it: how often is the mother the enforcer in a married parental relationship, and how often is the father the one who is tender and lenient and eternally compassionate? Single mothers tend to try to be both, but no one can achieve this. The overall effect is that boys are less able to move into the powerful, masculine energy thant makes them strong, capable men who can take care of business.

Materialism = Isolation

Many African-American households are caught up in another kind of dichotomy: on the one hand, there's poverty, trying to make ends meet against all odds; and on the other hand, there's an incredibly powerful materialism. Televisions, cars, computers, video games, designer clothing all take on an importance beyond that of family time or family unity.

We can't remedy lack of parenting time and skill by buying things for our children. On the contrary: every time a family buys a new TV, it creates a climate of isolation. Materialism has the effect of separating family members. With small children, TV and toys easily become mother substitutes, and most TV and toys teach all the wrong things.

If Junior has a TV in his room, or video games, or his own computer, he isn't going to spend family time.

When I was growing up, we had one TV, and we had to take the time and energy to negotiate what was watched on that TV. We learned how to negotiate, how to resolve conflict. This doesn't happen when children are isolated from one another and from parents who work all day and come home tired and stressed, and have no energy left for constructive interaction with their children.

Raising Our Girls Up Right

The problems of African-American families are at the root of the problems of African-American communities. A lot can be done to help these communities, but if parents don't get on track with their children, nothing else will solve the problems of violence, splintered families, young black men being incarcerated, and young black women carrying on the tradition of single motherhood. Boys must be taught to father and to be men; girls must be taught to be strong enough to resist the temptations of sex without commitment.

Although girls are wired to nurture and care for the home, they can use their early years to learn as much as they can in school, to educate their minds, and to learn how to be contributing members of the community—whether that is through family life, professional life, or a combination of both.

Girls need to be taught that mothering is a worthwhile occupation. Mothering has been shuttled to the bottom of the list of important things women do in the world, and this is an outrageous travesty. We need our girls to believe that birthing and raising children is one of the most valuable things they can do for their community and for the world. We need to convey to them that parenting is an art and a science and worthy of all of their best efforts. Sure, a lot of it is custodial—laundry, cooking, cleaning—but most days, it's also great fun and a great challenge with unparalleled rewards. This is particularly true for women who are part of a cohesive clan, which I will address in more detail in Chapter Eight.

It's okay to let our men take care of us. As it is, African-American women are going out and taking jobs away from African-American men. The rising tide of black women in the workforce has effectively castrated black men. If women are so independent and self-supporting, what do we need men for? Do we discard them once they've served their purposes as sperm donors? No—we need each other's support. Let's let the men go out and work to support their families, and they won't feel so inclined to get into trouble with the law. They'll feel vital, needed, necessary in the community again.

I became a clinician after a friend of mine committed suicide in the late 1980s. This friend was hugely successful in the work world, had burst through the "glass ceiling" and then some. Still, she was suffering so much inside that she elected to end her own life. I wanted to understand how that could have been. My studies in psychology school helped me to see what had happened to her, but it was not until I grasped the difficulty of being a 'career woman' who also is trying to raise a family and maintain a marriage that I fully understood what she had gone through. It's hard, it's really hard, and we have to prepare our daughters for that as they enter the work world and family life.

Good mothers make a good community. When we lost the nosy neighbor, we lost our best source of community protection. If you'll forgive my nostalgia, I'll harken back to my own childhood again: every mother was home during the day, tending to the house and doing the chores, and they kept an eye on the whole neighborhood, especially on the children. Then, in the 1970s, the whole "latchkey kid" phenomenon took hold, and kids started coming home to empty houses. Instead of interacting with their mothers over a plate of homemade cookies, they sat in front of TV and ate junk food.

This brings me to another point: the terrible problem of obesity in our community. Although overweight and obesity are serious issues across all races, it's worst in African-Americans, who seem especially vulnerable to becoming obese. We are also more likely to get Type 2 diabetes, high blood pressure, and heart disease than people of other races. Part of it is the food we consider to be our cultural birthright—if it's fried or covered in gravy, it's probably soul food—but a lot more can be attributed to the way we've been feeding our children junk food instead of fresh food for the last generation or so, and letting them sit in front of TV instead of exercising.

If we are obese as a race, it's the fault of the women who shop for their households. If black children are angry at their mothers, we need to accept that their anger is justified. Mothers: if you open up your sugar canister every morning in the guise of breakfast and send your child off to school with an air kiss, and then you tell him to come home to an empty house, do you really expect your child not to feel angry? Your child needs you there, today, every day, until he is a man or she is a woman.

Girls today are so drawn to a complete focus on getting and holding the attention of males who are—let's face it—undeserving. It's time to go back to the way it was when I was a girl: young men need to face the obstacle of *earning* the love of women, instead of having girls throw themselves at them. It's a ridiculous double standard right now: girls are told that they can do or be whatever they like in the world, and yet they are encouraged by the media to focus on their bodies and their sexuality to the exclusion of all else. They get the message that they are nothing without a man, and that they should take whatever man pays attention to them.

Don't think I am saying that women don't need men. We do. But we need *real* men, men who can take care of us, who can be loving and kind and supportive, who are willing to work hard, who will value us, who can help us to raise our children right—not gangbangers or felons or rapists or a man who would abandon the children he has fathered because some other honey has caught his eye.

Girls need a lot of help to navigate these confusing issues, and the best way to do that is to be *in their business and in their lives, all the time*. Boys, on the other hand, need to be taught how to be the kind of men women can have successful marriages and families with.

How can parents achieve this when they're off at work for much of the day? It isn't easy, but strengthening our communities will be a good start. When I was raising my own daughter, everyone knew everyone in our little town, and as soon as she did anything questionable, I knew about it.

Girls also must be shown repeatedly that the images that are absolutely everywhere in the media—particularly, the ones of barely dressed young black women who are obviously ready and willing for anything, and who gain the attentions of rich gangsta rappers—are not their reality, and that those women are not to be emulated. This can be difficult for mothers who are still girls themselves, who are still caught up in that imagery themselves, who feel they have to compete with their daughters, who wear tighter clothes and more makeup than their daughters and are caught up in the culture of drugs and promiscuous behavior.

Good parenting is not parenting that keeps children happy. Good parenting is not what is easiest on the parents. Good parenting is parenting that raises up an adult who is disciplined, motivated, and responsible. It is parenting that not only creates adults who can support a thriving, loving, and successful community, but that creates adults who know how to parent.

Keys to Productive Parenting

Parents need to cope with their own traumas—with whatever stands in the way of becoming adults themselves. Improving their parenting skills can't wait until this is done, however. Dealing with trauma is, as you'll find throughout the rest of this book, an ongoing process. Children need better parenting *right now,* and there are ways for parents who are still struggling with the lack of support they themselves suffered to improve their parenting skills.

Today, in a family that's struggling to make ends meet, mothers have no choice but to work. But we have to find ways to keep our communities connected. We have to take the initiative to know all that is going on in our children's lives—staying involved in their schools, with the parents of their friends and the friends of their friends.

Try to arrange help from a family member or family friend so that children don't come home to an empty house, so that they can have a nourishing snack after school. Or, if there are after-school programs available where your child can do homework or engage in sports or arts activities, send your children there while you're working.

Don't use TV as a babysitter. Strictly limit the time children can watch and keep track of what they're watching. And do everything within your power to be at home with your children when they are very young—from birth to preschool age. If you can't, try to work in a place with on-site daycare, or send your child to the home of a female family member: a grandmother, an aunt.

Parents always benefit from understanding the cognitive developmental stages children go through. Often, problems arise because parents expect too much or too little of their children, and knowing how children think and perceive at any given age helps parents to adjust their expectations. Our role as parents is not to control our children (as the authoritarian view would have us believe), or to be our children's best friends (as some single mothers, lonesome and dependent on their kids, might wish). It is to guide and assist them in their development.

If you've been doing things in a very different way than described throughout the rest of this chapter, don't let it discourage you. No parent does everything right, and most of us do a lot of things wrong. The important things are to always try to do our best; to take responsibility when we make a mistake; and to continually educate ourselves about how to better parent our children.

Children's Developmental Stages: Brief Overview

Birth to age one. Children in this age group learn through their senses and through the use of their own motor skills. They explore their environments through what they see, hear, and touch. This is why it is so important to give infants and toddlers plenty of sensory stimulation.

I'm not talking about those brightly colored, costly "learning toys" with their blinking lights and electronic noises, or of the videos that have become so popular; those toys aren't of much use unless a human being is using them to engage the child's attention. The most important source of stimulation for an infant or toddler is his mother. In holding and caressing him, in smiling and talking to him, in engaging him in play, and in carrying him around with her throughout the day, the mother is giving that child all the stimulation he needs.

A child this young is definitely not ready to be separated from its mother for any length of time. Mothers who breastfeed exclusively are especially bound to their infants, and while some would regard this as a negative thing—as being "tied down" to their babies 24/7—it's really Mother Nature's way of trying to ensure that the mother stays with her baby pretty much all the time.

A school of thought known as *attachment parenting* simplifies the matter of parenting babies under the age of one. Attachment parenting holds that a baby needs to be held or in contact with a warm, responsive human body as much as possible, until she's able to move about confidently on her own.

Following a healthy birth, mother and baby immediately bond with one another, and remaining in physical proximity for most of the first nine months of the child's life enables that attachment to fluorish and deepen. Attachment parenting promotes the use of baby slings and other types of carriers (see the Resources section for how to get a baby sling—some of which are modeled after those that are used by African women) and nursing the baby on demand (whenever the infant's cues indicate to Mom that it's feeding time). Many parents who subscribe to the attachment parenting school of thought also "co-sleep" with their infant or young child, nursing during the night if needed without having to get up.

Children who are parented this way are almost invariably happier, more contented, and less demanding—because their demands are being met without them having to cry out for them. Of course, it's hard to do this if you have to go to work and put your child in daycare, but if at all possible, try to be with your infant and toddler during these important months. For more on attachment parenting, check out *The Baby Book* by Dr. William Sears.

The bond created during this time won't make your child overly attached to you, as some might fear. It fulfills the child's need for early nurturing and closeness with Mom, so that when it's time to venture out into the world as a preschooler and beyond, she'll be secure in the knowledge that she is safe—that you will be there when you need her. Spending lots of time with your infant and toddler will help you to parent him intuitively. You'll know his cues and his problems and the games he loves to play.

The Baby that Won't Quit Crying

A baby that cries often can be enough to drive even the most patient mother to distraction. Some parents are shocked at their own inability to comfort their babies. They've checked the diaper, they've tried to feed, they've examined him from crown to sole for "boo-boos," but he will not stop screaming. Now what?

Parents who were raised by authoritative parents themselves might feel that they should not spoil the child, and that attending to him when he's crying so much would do just that. Or, worse, parents who were subjected to abuse when they were children might lose control and become abusive under these circumstances.

Any child under the age of two who is crying is just trying to tell you that she needs something from you. They are not capable of manipulation at this young an age. You can't give too much attention or love to a child this young; it all goes towards strengthening the child's security and self-esteem.

Even if the child seems inconsolable, simply hold him tight. Accept that your child needs to cry sometimes. Encourage him: "That's good. Yes, have a good cry. You're doing fine. You're doing great." Give up on trying to make him stop—as long as you're sure that all his needs are met and that he doesn't need the attentions of a doctor. Cry with him if you feel like it.

> If you don't feel you can be with your inconsolable baby without taking your frustration out on her by shaking her, hitting her, or screaming at her, don't hesitate to walk away. Leave the baby to cry while you collect yourself or get someone in to help you out.

Age one to two. Children who are on the move but have little or no impulse control can be as frustrating as a baby who won't stop crying. Everything in sight goes in their mouths; they dash into the street without warning while on a walk; they break things and mess up the house with total glee.

Keep in mind during this challenging time that your toddler can't understand *why* she shouldn't do something. Her impulses to explore are more powerful than her desire to please you or to do what she's told. She isn't misbehaving, she's just not in control. The parents have to begin to teach her how to control herself during this time. Start creating boundaries, but keep it as simple as possible: "no, don't touch—ouch!" when little Daniel goes for the stove, or "no, yuck, don't eat—bad for Janelle" when she tries to eat a handful of salt.

Punishing a child this young does virtually no good. They just don't get it. Instead of yelling at or threatening a child who repeatedly goes back for more toy boat fun in the toilet, distract him with another activity. Don't give in, though, even if he refuses to be distracted. This is the beginning of boundary-setting. Once you've said no to something, don't give in, because your child will learn that if he persists, he'll eventually get you to give him what he wants.

Don't take saying "no" lightly, because you're going to have to insist, in order to be consistent with your child. Choose your battles carefully. Set up your home so that you can avoid saying "no" as much as possible. If you don't want your child to play with flour because it makes a mess, think about the value of the play experience and weigh it against some time with the broom and dustpan. Create situations where you can be positive instead of negative.

If your child continually challenges you past the point where you think he should have gotten the message, try a "time-out" in a playpen. Don't, however, send your child out of the room or otherwise isolate her. She needs to know that even when she misbehaves, she is still safe, still loved.

What About Spanking?

In most African-American households, parents will still whack a child good if he doesn't do as he's told. A firm swat on the bottom is appropriate if—and only if—you're absolutely sure that he knows what you want from him (and a one-year-old should be able to catch on to this); if you believe that his safety is at risk because of what he insists upon doing; and if there's no alternative way to get him out of harm's way.

Let's say your 18-month-old girl is walking alongside you in the market. As you wait in line to buy your groceries, your arms too full to pick her up, she tries to dart out the front door onto the busy sidewalk, which borders on a traffic-filled street. "Stay with Mama—not safe to run outside!" you tell her, but as soon as you let go of her arm she's off again. You catch her and bring her back, and when you release her to get your wallet out, she starts to scoot away from you again. Now's the time to give her a quick swat on the rear—not hard enough to really hurt (especially if she's wearing diapers) but hard enough to get her attention. Then, tell her: "Mommy told you not to run away," and hold onto her hand.

Sibling rivalry that blossoms into violence can also be dealt with this way in children who are still elementary school age or younger. If children start to fight one another and you can't get them to stop, a smack on the rear for both parties will break up the melee quickly.

Preschool years. Here are Dr. Hicks-Ray's keys to parenting toddlers and preschoolers well: be consistent; be loving; be firm; be positive; and be *the adult.*

Do your absolute best to remain calm. Small children thrive on all kinds of attention, and as they get older they are trying to find out how to control their universe—including the people who populate it. If they know they can get your goat and make you furious, it might just be worth whatever punishment ends up being meted out to them.

Don't be so concerned with being right all the time. Raising kids is about a lot more than having things done your way. If you see parenting as a test of your ability to control your children, you'll really miss out on all your children can teach you. Authoritarian parents teach children to do things their way, but they sacrifice teaching children to think for themselves. Remember, we have to give children the tools to discipline themselves and motivate themselves, not to always look to others for discipline and motivation.

Elementary school, middle school, and the teen years. If you've done most things right up to this point, your children will probably stay out of serious trouble once they become old enough to get into it. You need to continue to watch your children like a hawk, however, and to be ready for anything. Even a "good kid" can get into a world of trouble. A kid that's already been in trouble needs plenty of support—and sometimes professional help—to get back on track. Sometimes the job is too much for parents, and there's no shame in seeking out help when a child is acting out.

A lot of hazardous issues that were never a concern for me in my own childhood or for my daughter in hers are coming up for children of elementary school age. They're exposed to sexuality and violence that they are completely unprepared to deal with, developmentally and physically. Girls and boys as young as nine are having sexual relations and dabbling with alcohol and drugs. Many are maturing early, with girls starting their menses and developing breasts much sooner than girls of previous generation. Like the one-year-old who can walk long before she has any concept of where she can do so safely, these girls who develop prematurely have no idea how to deal with womanhood or the dangers and joys it can bring. Teenaged girls need a strong foundation in the home to help them resist becoming sexual too soon.

I can't reiterate enough that parents need to be in their children's business and in their lives. Stay involved. Make sure you know where your children are and what they're up to. Limit their TV, computer game, and phone time and keep them focused on their studies, extracurricular activities (sports, art, music) and on their family, church, and community connections. Control and track Internet access. When you do allow them to watch TV, use it as an opportunity to talk about issues that are dealt with in age-appropriate programs. Engage them in conversation. Help them to explore things that interest them. Do things together as a family.

If your children suddenly clam up completely, chances are good that there's something you need to know about. Don't be afraid to nag them until the truth comes out. They'll thank you for it later. Be available to hear whatever's on their minds, and do your best to be non-judgemental and non-punitive, so that they don't feel afraid to open up to you about sensitive issues such as sex, drugs, and violence.

Model good relationship skills for your children. If you're not sure how to do this—if you and your mate argue often and can't seem to resolve your problems—see if you can get some couples counseling. (I'll tell you more about this in Chapter Nine.) Read together; a child who reads is a child who succeeds.

Discipline is crucial during these years. You will need to be consistent, firm, fair, and available. Require that your children respect their elders, and model respect in the way that you treat your children and your mate. Teach children how to treat people of the opposite sex, and what can be expected from them. Stay a step ahead of them at all times.

They need to know that they must do as you tell them (but that as long as they breach the subject in a respectful way, they can protest what they are being told they must do); that they must never lie; and that they earn privileges (time to watch TV, playing computer games, going out with friends) by doing what is required of them, including chores and schoolwork.

When my daughter began elementary school, I began to give her the option of taking totally free "mental health" days off from school. She got to choose the days, and she got to do whatever she liked with that day. As she increased her level of responsibility she got more days off; for example, when she was in fifth grade, she got to take two mental health days, and when she got good grades that year she was given three days in sixth grade. This taught her that perfect attendance does not equal perfect production; that taking time off to refuel is okay, that she doesn't have to be Superwoman. She was valedictorian of her senior high school class and president of her junior and senior high school classes.

Begin teaching children about money as soon as they're able to add, subtract, divide, and multiply. Talk about how it's made, how it's spent, how to keep track of it. An allowance is a good tool for this. Talk to them about the power of advertising and how to see when they are being manipulated into spending money on something they don't really need. Continually reiterate that *things* are less important than *people* and the relationships you have with them.

Feed Your Children Right, Body and Soul

Women are the nurturers of the community. In most households, the woman does the shopping and the cooking. It's her responsibility to teach the children about healthy eating, to set an example, and to prepare healthy meals for them. In Chapter Seven, you'll learn some guidelines for a healthful diet that kids will actually eat—once they've gotten over cravings for addictive junk foods.

Eating junk has influence on more than body weight. It has been found that foods loaded with artificial coloring, sugar, and artificial flavors actually affect brain function and behavior. Children with serious behavior problems have been cured with diets free of these ingredients, and school programs that bring nutritious, natural foods to children have reliably improved test scores.

Nourish children's souls by helping them to deal with the pain that will inevitably come up in their lives: not by telling them to get over it, or by trying to make them feel better, but by sitting with them and letting them experience it fully, until it's played itself out. Allow your children to cry, be frustrated, be angry, be confused as readily as you allow them to smile, laugh, be happy, be intelligent.

Teach them that there's room for all of it. In tribal life in more primitive times, rituals enabled people to work through their pain, but in modern times we don't have that outlet.

Church and spiritual study can help a lot with this, and you can work through some of your own pain in the company of those most precious people in your life: your children.

Chapter Seven

Holistic Healing: Setting the Foundation

Lately, I've had occasion to visit a number of large cities on the East coast. I noticed a disturbing trend in inner-city areas. Police presence has had some success in keeping those who deal illegal drugs off of the street corners, but now, every corner has a 24-hour drugstore—a perfectly legal place of business, open all night, where hundreds of different consciousness-altering substances can be bought cheaply.

I'm talking about over-the-counter drugs, yes: sedatives, cold medicine, diet pills, cough syrup, and a lot of other chemicals considered to be perfectly good medicine. And, of course, cigarettes. But I'm also talking about the items that line all of the other aisles—particularly, junk food: sodas, candy, chips, cake, cookies, sugary fruit drinks.

Most people don't think of these items as consciousness-altering, but science has proven that junk food is addicting, that it acts in a manner similar to the opiates made in the brain. It is very commonly used to mask and hide from pain—a fact that is painfully obvious, due to the extraordinary number of overweight and obese people walking the Earth.

According to data from the Department of Health and Human Services, in the year 2001, 61 percent of Americans aged 20 or older was overweight, and a quarter of Americans are obese. In a study published in the *North Carolina Medical Journal* in 2002, it was found that in a group of 1200 children aged 11 to 14, 32.4 percent were overweight and 16.4 percent were obese. Of the African-American children involved in this study, 54 percent of females and 45 percent of males were overweight, and more than half of these children were categorized as obese.

When I see a grossly overweight person, I see *pain.* Not just physical pain, although aches and pains and joint problems are more common in people who carry around a lot of extra pounds. Excess fat is pain made flesh.

When people overeat to the point of allowing themselves to become disfigured and imprisoned within a body that can't run, jump, play, or dance as bodies are made to, there is much more than gluttony at work. Even people who are moderately overweight may be eating to mask pain, and they happen to be lucky enough—or vain enough—to not let things spiral out of control.

African-Americans and Rates of Chronic Disease

There is no shortage of pain in the inner-city African-American community, and these folks spend millions of dollars trying to protect themselves against it. Better we should eat doughnuts than shoot heroin, but just because the doughnuts are the lesser of two evils doesn't mean that they're harmless.

We medicate ourselves with material things, too: cars, big-screen TVs, toys, clothes, makeup. This is also a problem. It also masks what must be acknowledged in order for trauma's wounds to be healed. But in this chapter, I'd like to focus on changing the foods we eat so that we can be clear in mind and body. I'll address materialism more closely in Chapter Ten (hiphop/rap).

African-Americans are, overall, more likely to to be obese, and to have heart attacks, high blood pressure, adult-onset (type 2) diabetes, and cancer than are people of other races. We die younger. We are, in the words of Elijah Saunders, M.D., cardiologist at University of Maryland Medical Center, "significantly more likely to die from the consequences of high blood pressure than the general public." Almost 40 percent of African-American adults suffer from some kind of heart disease, and 13 percent have type 2 diabetes. Thirty-two percent of the people who are on dialysis due to kidney failure (a result of uncontrolled high blood pressure) are African-American.

Income inequity has a great deal to do with the fact that African-Americans get sicker and die younger than whites: women whose families make $10,000 or less per year are three times more likely to die of heart disease and almost three times as likely to die of diabetes than women whose families make $25,000 or more. So do differences in education: men who have fewer than 12 years of education are more than twice as likely to die of chronic disease (including heart disease and diabetes). African-Americans are more likely to smoke cigarettes, consume too much alcohol, and avoid exercise when compared with whites.

Poverty has a good deal to do with the differences between health outcomes in whites and African-Americans, but it doesn't explain all of those differences. In a 1996 study published in the *New England Journal of Medicine,* African-American women who lived to the age of 15 in Harlem had about the same chance of making it to age 65 as women in India (65 percent)—a much poorer country with much higher incidence of infectious diseases. Life expectancy for African-American males is roughly equivalent to life expectancy in El Salvador, despite the income of the average African-American male being five times that of the average El Salvadorean male.

Poverty is relative, not absolute. As you'll see later in this chapter, there is more to racial and social inequality than differences in paychecks. Earning more dollars would most certainly help African-Americans, but better health won't come to us if we're not feeling secure, if we're not part of a unified clan, if we're not living our lives as though we are important to ourselves and to the others in our communities.

Poor people can't afford health insurance—neither can the middle-class, nowadays—and they are only half as likely to see a doctor for a health problem than someone with high income. The poor rely on emergency room care, which they only use when they are desperately ill with a problem that could have been remedied much more easily if it had been attended to early on.

Disparity between the healthiness of African-Americans and whites is about pain, and about feeling like there's no way to get ahead in the world. Hopelessness and low status both have detrimental effects on health.

Some interesting research suggests a link between social status and chronic disease. When a person (or animal) has low social status, he is more likely to develop hypertension. When a person feels that she has little or no control over her life—for example, if that person holds a job where she is always being told what to do and how to act and rarely or never gets an opportunity to exert control over others—she is more likely to die an early death.

In this context, it makes sense that traumatized people who have felt helpless would turn around and do violence to others. It is a self-preservation instinct, an intrinsic understanding that if you don't get some control over someone or something, you're not going to make it, you're going to be phased out, because you're not necessary in the grand scheme of things.

Fortunately, the possession or lack of control or social status is not something that is absolute. Changing your way of looking at your life is a much better way of gaining control than trying to smash others to grab control away from them. There's always going to be someone bigger and stronger than you, waiting to smash you down once you think you're the top dog. A peaceful mindset, a non-competitive and a non-violent way of looking at the world, will bring you that feeling of control.

I don't mean to say that we should not be competitive. Competition is a source of energy and fun, and it is a powerful motivator. We need to learn how to compete better, more fairly. We need to maintain the rules of good sportsmanship, and we need to teach those rules to our children and expect them from each other. Once upon a time, we could compete without killing each other, and we can do so again.

According to Michael Marmot, who researches links between social inequality and disease, the so-called "diseases of affluence" —which are caused by high-calorie, high-fat diets and lack of exercise—are actually far more prevalent in the poor than they are in the wealthy. When you think about it, this is really incontrovertible. If you walk through an inner city, you see a lot more heavy people than you see if you walk through an upscale shopping district. People with greater financial security can afford to eat healthy, and they can afford to educate themselves about how to make healthy choices. They can also see a therapist to help them deal with stress and trauma instead of sitting on a couch with a friend to eat a whole bag of barbecue potato chips with a liter bottle of fruit punch to chase it down. They can join a gym and actually have time to go every day.

Obesity is at its peak in the general population. If there is any more obvious symptom of unhealthy lifestyle choices, I haven't yet seen it. Being fat raises our risk of all kinds of disease and decreases our quality of life. It also works the other way: when someone is fat, you can pretty much assume that they got that way because of unhappiness—either their own or that of the people who raised them.

Most heartbreaking of all is the state of the health of many African-American children who are raised in poor or middle-class homes. When I see an obese six-year-old waddling down the street with his parents, who are usually also obese, I want to cry. That child is going to struggle against that weight for the rest of his days. The children of African-American parents are more at risk for obesity and suffer more from asthma than white children. Living in polluted inner cities increases a child's chances of developing asthma or being exposed to high levels of lead, which accumulate in their bodies and decrease their intelligence. In the suburbs, increasing reliance on cars prevents children (and adults) from getting the exercise they need.

Cancer rates are also higher in African-American men than in their white counterparts. According to SEER Cancer Statistics 2003, the cancer rate of black men is 697 per 100,000, compared with 556 per 100,000 for white men. They are 1.4 times more likely to die from cancer, most often from lung, prostate, colorectal, or pancreatic cancers. (White women have slightly higher cancer rates than African-American women. Keep in mind, however, that white women also have better access to testing and treatment than African-American women, and cancer is often not detected until it has become advanced.)

Trauma and Physical Health

Let's top all of this off by revisiting the physiological consequences of trauma. Post-traumatic stress can make you physically ill. It alters levels of hormones that make a big difference in a person's state of health. So does unrelenting, inescapable stress.

This is especially true of children, and childhood abuse often takes a toll on physical health right up on into adulthood. One study found that women who were subjected to childhood sexual or physical abuse were significantly more likely to develop chronic fatigue syndrome, bladder problems, chronic headaches (including migraines), asthma, diabetes, and heart disease. Many other studies have revealed similar results.

The physical consequences of chronic or acute trauma can last for years or even for a lifetime. Relieving trauma-related physical symptoms necessitates dealing with the trauma in therapy and within a caring community. But the changes that are accomplished there won't take hold, won't be complete, without attention to healing and caring for the physical body. I'm talking about a healthful diet (which may not be what you think), exercise, and a mind-body practice like meditation or yoga that will defuse the physical changes that come from being in a state of hyperarousal. I also think that herbs, Bach flower remedies, and nutritional supplements have a place in the holistic healing of trauma-related physical symptoms.

Caring for the whole self in this way has many rewards aside from simply dealing with trauma. It will help you to break away from food addictions. It will help you to value yourself more—to show you how treating yourself right means feeding yourself right. It will help you to parent better, to show you that giving your kids junk food isn't a loving act, no matter how much they enjoy it. It will help you to take a proactive role in caring for your own health.

Feed Yourself (and Your Family) Right

How much is your health worth to you? How about the health of your children? What are you really worth to yourself? Are you only worth a $1.19 bottle of sugary juice drink from the corner store? *I'm* worth more than that. I'm worth freshly squeezed juice that I make at home with a juice extractor. I make a small glass—there are no extra-large, big-gulp fresh-squeezed juices going into my body—and it's very nourishing. I know you are worth at least that, yourself.

There is a mindset that buying the cheapest possible food is a good thing. I've seen mothers buying expired food at the dollar store, thinking that this is a good way to save a few dollars—but not thinking of the eventual cost to the health of themselves and their families. If there is anything worth investing in, it's eating well.

I watched my father die of cancer. People I know have died slow deaths from diabetes and heart disease. I wouldn't wish any of it on my worst enemy, much less myself or my child, but many are feeding themselves and their families in a way that hugely increases their risk of ending up in that position as their lives come to an end. People live their lives eating junk and smoking cigarettes and exposing themselves to all kinds of toxic hazards, then they spend hundreds of thousands of dollars in the last months of their lives, in and out of the hospital, desperately trying to buy just a month or two more time. Wouldn't you rather put up the money up front—invest it in a healthy diet and consistent exercise program?

Of course, those who have insurance have, in the past, seen most or all of these end-of-life disease expenses covered. Today's climate is very different. Insurance premiums are too high for more than half of people to pay, and coverage is spotty at best even when we have insurance. We are increasingly unable to handle the risk of incurring huge hospital bills at the end of our lives.

You don't need a big-screen TV or a new couch or a new outfit if you can't afford to give your family and yourself fresh, wholesome food. You can't afford to *not* eat well.

We worry too much about not having enough food. Most of us could stand to eat far less than we do. A diet that's lower in total calories has been found to extend lifespan and prevent chronic disease. Let yourself get hungry once in a while rather than feeling like you have to have a larder totally stocked with snacks and convenience foods. It won't hurt you to do this, and it won't hurt your children, either. Spend your money on good food, even if this means eating less food. The supersizing trend is killing us. All-you-can-eat buffets are making us fatter than any generation that has come before.

The African-American Diet: A Historical Perspective

According to research from the U.S. Department of Agriculture (USDA), the diet of the typical African-American is of "particularly poor quality." Our culture is very strongly tied to food. This is the case with most races who have a history of persecution and segregation: food becomes part of the glue that holds us together, a source of comfort and community. That relationship with food can easily become self-destructive when too much of it is available, and when so much of it is empty calories full of sugar, unhealthful fats, and artificial ingredients.

In the 15th and 16th centuries, before we came to America on the slave ships, we ate foods such as cassava (a type of tuber, like potatoes), corn, chile peppers, peanuts, tomatoes, and pumpkin. Africans evolved for millennia on a plant-rich diet with some nuts and meat. Slave diets added pork and pork fat, chicken, sausage, sweet potatoes, rice, leafy greens, fish, black-eyed peas, okra, grits, peas, and squash. Our ancestors in America were adept at adapting their Old World recipes to New World foods.

Overall, this is a pretty healthy diet, and slaves worked long hours and bore and raised many children while living on these foods. They did, however, have to make the best they could with what their masters' families threw away. They found ways to make the worst cuts of meat palatable, adding fat and sweetener to try to get past the unsavory taste. Soul food is the modern take on this kind of culinary creativity. African-Americans still do this today.

Today, you're likely to see fried chicken, barbecue, corn bread, sweet potato pie, macaroni and cheese, many kinds of chips and dips, and fruit-flavored drinks at an African-American gathering. The collards are still there, but their nutrition can't make up for the preponderance of greasy, fatty, and sugary foods. Fast food is a staple of American families, and the supersizing of fast-food meals has doubled and tripled the amount of food they eat at a sitting.

Eating healthy doesn't have to mean giving up on soul food. A healthy diet just gets rid of all of the processed junk and focuses on fresh foods: vegetables, whole grains, beans, peas, nuts, and lean meats.

Eat Like Your Ancestors

Diets come and go; there's the low-fat, the high-protein, the "negative calorie" diet, the grapefruit diet, the diets where you subsist on sugary meal replacement shakes, and on and on and on. Many of us watched as Oprah lost and gained and lost and gained again on these kinds of diets. In a world where so many people are fat and trying to lose weight, just about any fool with the resources to do so can make a killing selling weight loss plans, whether they work or not.

The truth of the matter is that eating right is not rocket science. It's not *theoretically* difficult, although it may be *practically* difficult. The secret is to adhere as closely as possible to the diets of the people from which we are descended. I'm not talking about your parents, or even their parents; I'm talking about prehistory, the roots of humankind. Africans were, after all, the first human beings. All others are descended from those first Africans.

Why would you want to eat like your earliest ancestors? Why should you eat meat and greens instead of macaroni and cheese? Because your genetic makeup has a lot to do with the foods that are ideal for your body. Your genes are strikingly similar to the genes of your primitive ancestors. They've been passed down through generations without much change. It takes millions of years for really significant changes to take place within the genome.

Genetic change definitely hasn't happened over the past 200 years, during which enormous changes took place in the typical diet. In only the span of a couple of centuries, human beings went from eating whole foods from the earth and from livestock that they often killed and dressed themselves to living on highly processed, preservative—and sugar-loaded junk.

Your genes provide instructions within each of your cells, driving every function of your body. They aren't exactly "blueprints," as they're often described; there is a certain amount of flexibility in their expression, depending on environmental factors. For example: many of us have been led to believe that being overweight has something to do with our genes. "If it's in my genes," we think, "it's not my fault. I'm just made to be fat, and there's nothing I can do about it!" The truth is that yes, some of us are more genetically geared to gain weight, but there's a lot we can do to control that tendency. Just because we can't be a perfect size six doesn't mean we should let ourselves balloon out of control. Same with heart disease, digestive problems, diabetes, and high blood pressure: just because others in your family have had these problems, you don't have to have them—at least not as early in life or as severely.

We've got to acknowledge our responsibility to take care of our own health—to maintain the temple of our bodies, to sustain ourselves with healthful foods rather than the junk that might help us to stave off pain temporarily, but that stays on our bodies in the form of extra fat for a lot longer. I know this has been said countless times before, but we must love ourselves first, because if we love ourselves we won't feed ourselves so much garbage.

Another important part of changing our diets is to change the way our children eat. African-American children are dealing with enough without having to also deal with being overweight, overstimulated, and overly susceptible to catching every bug that goes through their schools from eating poorly. I see children walking to catch the schoolbus in the morning, eating bags of corn chips and drinking fruit punch. I know they have access to fast food and sodas in school, because struggling public schools are turning more and more to deals with fast food and soda companies to try to make ends meet. Just as we teach our kids how to parent, we must also teach them how to eat.

According to Peter D'Adamo, the naturopath who developed the dietary plan outlined in the *Eat Right For Your Type* books, your genetic makeup is best reflected by your blood type. Blood type represents the presence of certain *antibodies*—immune factors that affect many aspects of body functions. It follows that if you eat foods that react poorly with your blood type, you're more likely to gain weight and feel generally unwell.

Type O is the original blood type. In the earliest days of humanity, everyone was blood type O. We lived on a hunter-gatherer diet in those days. D'Adamo's theory tells us that Type Os are made to eat lots of protein in the form of lean red meat, along with lots of vegetables and relatively few carbohydrates. Dairy products tend to disagree with Type Os, and grains, bread, and legumes (including peas, beans, and peanuts) also don't agree with this blood type.

What does eating the wrong foods do to a Type O? D'Adamo theorizes that weight gain and low energy will result from a diet that emphasizes foods not tailored to our blood types.

If you're a type A, a type AB, or a type B, there are other dietary guidelines D'Adamo advises you to follow. These other blood types evolved as civilization evolved, to adapt to the changing diets brought about because of agriculture and the domestication of animals. For example: type As seem better adapted to vegetarian diets that include lots of whole grains and legumes; type Bs and type ABs seem to thrive on diets somewhere in the middle.

D'Adamo's theories aren't exactly based in a great deal of hard science—although he has done research on the subject for more than 15 years, piggybacking on his naturopath father's 30 years of study on blood type and diet—but they make very good sense, and they work well for a lot of people. If you're interested in finding out more, I recommend that you look at the book he wrote with Catherine Whitney, *Eat Right 4 Your Type: The Individualized Diet Solution to Staying Healthy, Living Longer & Achieving Your Ideal Weight* (G.P. Putnam's Sons,New York, NY: 1997).

Whether or not you subscribe to the blood type theory of eating right, there are a few hard, fast guidelines to follow if you want to feed yourself and your family in a way that will promote their health and keep their weight down. It is now understood that diet plays a major role in creating health—and, conversely, can play a major role in creating disease. Foods dramatically affect our moods, our ability to think clearly, and our ability to pay attention. They affect the function of our immune systems, the health of our skin (acne has been linked with poor diet in several studies), and the menstrual health of women. Year after year of eating poorly set us up to develop obesity, diabetes, heart disease, and cancer. This is not speculation; it is scientific fact.

Children who are believed to suffer from ADHD, hyperactivity, or other learning problems often make huge improvements when artificial flavorings, colorings, and allergenic foods are removed from their diets. Although most of these additives have been called safe by the government agencies responsible for testing their safety, they are best avoided. You don't need them, and there's sufficient evidence that they can be bad for some people to merit your finding other foods to eat.

Think about Jesus, or Buddha, or Allah, or whoever you choose to make the centerpiece of your religious worship. Think about how these great men ate. They didn't eat fluorescent-colored bits of hydrogenated oil and sugar (which is what most candies are made of); they didn't pull up to a fast-food window and order super-sized, greasy meals. They ate food that came from nature.

They knew where their food had come from. That food had been grown in rich soil or grazed on grassy fields, not forced to grow in depleted ground through the use of chemical fertilizers or in a factory farm where they're dosed up on antibiotics and hormones just to keep them alive long enough to slaughter.

Your body, my body, they're just like the bodies of people who lived millennia ago. Why should we expect our bodies and minds to be able to function to their greatest potential when we don't even eat real food, when all the goodness has been processed out of everything we put in our mouths? It's astonishing, really, that human beings can function at all on the foods that just about everyone eats these days.

When the Creator designed the foods humans were made to eat, provisions were made to make those foods tasty and for those foods to give our bodies exactly what they need. Going back to those basic provisions is, in my opinion, the key to a healthy diet.

We tend to only use the parables that are convenient for us; while we might be willing to do unto others as we would have them do unto us, we all too often are not willing to treat *ourselves* right. We disrespect our bodies when we eat unnatural foods. And our bodies are retaliating by getting fat; our arteries are retaliating by constricting and clogging up with deposits of cholesterol. In the unluckiest of us, some of our cells transform into cancerous growths. Down to each and every cell, our bodies rebel by becoming insulin resistant.

Insulin resistance is the first step towards type 2 diabetes. This disease is epidemic across all races, but African-Americans get it more than others, and it is the sixth leading cause of death from disease in the developed world. We are approximately twice as likely to develop type 2 diabetes than are non-Hispanic whites. Black diabetics are significantly more likely to lose function in their kidneys and eyes than people of other races do when they become diabetic. Alarmingly, more and more children are developing a disease that has, until recently, been called *adult-onset diabetes.* African-American women of childbearing age are 50 to 80 percent more likely to develop gestational diabetes during pregnancy, a form of type 2 diabetes, and this increases her risk of developing type 2 diabetes again later in life, as well as increasing her chances of having a complicated and dangerous pregnancy.

The easiest way to explain insulin resistance is to look at it as the body revolting against constant onslaught of sugary, fatty foods. Each of our body cells needs glucose—the simplest form of sugar—to burn for fuel. Carbohydrates in our diet are broken down to glucose in the digestive system and absorbed into the bloodstream, and it is then transported throughout the body for use in individual cells. Insulin is like the doorman that opens the cellular "doors" to glucose and escorts it inside, where it can be metabolized.

When we become insulin resistant, the doorman starts to feel like he isn't getting paid enough to do this job, and he starts to take longer and longer breaks. Eventually he starts sneaking around the corner for a drink, and eventually he might decide to take off for good. Glucose begins to build up in the bloodstream, with nowhere to go. This leads to chronically high blood sugar, which is damaging to the blood vessels. Cells deprived of energy are forced to begin to burn fat instead of sugar, which might seem like a good thing—but it can cause a chemical imbalance in the body if done to excess, an imbalance called *ketosis*. Ketosis acidifies the body, and if it's allowed to go too far it leads to coma and death.

What causes insulin resistance? Almost to a person, insulin resistance only happens in people who are overweight. It's as though your body were saying, "OK, enough food already! We've got enough in storage to last a long time. No more sugar, thanks." Certain races seem more vulnerable because our bodies are geared to work best in a feast/famine mode. Over centuries of lean times alternating with periodic plenty, our bodies developed the ability to store lots of energy as fat when times are good, so that we can survive the lean times. In modern civilization, there isn't any famine, so we keep on packing on the pounds. This genetic predisposition to put plenty of food in storage in our bodies has long been an advantage for people of African descent, but it doesn't jive well with modern high-calorie, low-nutrition diets.

Insulin resistance and type 2 diabetes are preventable. Some are more vulnerable than others because of genetic predisposition, but if you eat a whole-foods diet without a lot of added sugar and you avoid bread, crackers, chips, cookies, cake, and other foods made of refined flour (and yes, that includes pasta), you can completely reverse them. Oh, and you also have to exercise—but more on that later.

My dietary dos and don'ts aren't hard to understand, but they will probably involve more time in the kitchen and more careful shopping at the store. I know that this is not easy, but it is more than worth the effort.

Following these guidelines will also involve calling a halt to using junk food to medicate pain or create community. If you feel that this is impossible for you, I recommend that you check into a twelve-step program that deals with food addiction. Clearing your head and heart through Overeaters Anonymous or a similar support program will make a big difference. Once you've done that, the rest will seem easy. You can find the Overeaters Anonymous website at www.oa.org/, or call them at (505) 891-2664 to find a meeting near you.

Your children may stage an outright rebellion if you suddenly take away those addictive treats they've grown used to having free access to. It's not possible to completely control what children eat, especially if they're teenagers. Not having unhealthy foods in the home will at least help them to experience something different, and if they insist on spending their own money on garbage, there's not a lot you can do about it. Let them see how slim, healthy, and balanced you become by eating well, and maybe they'll follow suit.

As an homage to all of those cute names for diet programs, I'd like to present my own as:

—Dr. Denyse's Diet Dos and Don'ts

Eat foods in a form that is as close as possible to the way the Creator made them.

Rice is from nature; packaged instant rice mixtures with seasoning packets aren't. A piece of baked chicken is from nature; chicken nuggets aren't. A bowl of cooked millet or spelt is from nature; a fluffy loaf of white bread is not. A piece of fresh, ripe fruit is from nature; a can full of sweetened chopped bits of fruit isn't. Poached eggs are from nature; a bowl of brightly colored, sweetened cereal isn't. There is no natural equivalent to cookies, cake, ice cream, doughnuts, chips, candy, or dip. Nothing in nature resembles fruit punch or soda.

Processing of foods removes their nutrients and fiber. Since nutrients are what give foods color and taste, food manufacturers replace them with sugar and unhealthy fats. The tastes and textures of these foods are strongly addictive and they are terrible for your health.

When word got out from the world of scientific research that high-fat, high-cholesterol diets might be to blame for the epidemics of obesity and heart disease, food manufacturers made a brilliant move: they started to make lots of "low-fat" and "fat-free" foods. These foods were marketed as healthy, but the truth is that they're just as processed as any other processed food. They may be fat-free, but they're generally loaded with artificial flavors and sugar to try to make up for the loss of the fat that has been removed. Don't be suckered into spending good money on these kinds of foods. You're better off having a modest portion of the real thing than you are having a huge portion of the unsatisfying fat-free alternative.

When you go to the grocery store, shop the produce section first instead of last, and stay out of those center aisles where the junk food and prepared foods live. Or, if you have a local farmer's market, shop there. Cook foods by steaming, broiling, poaching, or stir-frying with a small amount of oil. Use lots of herbs and spices to bring out foods' flavors instead of salt, sugar, and grease. It's as simple as that.

Living in the inner city may make this seem impossible. Access to fresh foods in urban areas can be slim to nonexistent. Residents of the inner city may find that fresh foods are inaccessible, that they would have to travel a long way in order to buy these foods. It's a whole lot easier to sit down to a fast-food burger and fries than it is to buy and prepare lean meat and fresh vegetables and fruits. I understand this, but we have to do whatever is necessary to start feeding ourselves and our families real food.

Grocery stores are now overwhelmingly located in suburban areas rather than inner cities. Even if they can get to a market that sells fresh vegetables and fruit, the prices of these foods may be prohibitive, and if they are on food stamp programs or WIC (Women, Infants, and Children) subsidies, they find that fresh foods are less emphasized than bread, cheese, and milk. (This is because the government is in the pocket of the processed food industry, but that's a story for another time.)

This so-called "grocery gap" is a major problem for many African-American families. In LA County, for example, the higher the concentration of people in a geographic area, the fewer supermarkets exist to serve them. In zip codes where zero to 10 percent of the households live below the federal poverty line, there are 2.26 times more supermarkets per household than in zip codes where more than 40 percent of families live in poverty. The higher the concentration of whites in a community, the greater the number of supermarkets.

Inner-city garden projects have sprung up in many metropolitan areas to help bring fresh foods to those who live there, but we've still got a long way to go.

How about organic foods? Doubtless, you're better off eating organic than not, but the cost of doing so is beyond the means of many, and finding organic produce, grains, meats, or dairy in the inner city is about as likely as finding a needle in a trash heap. If you can find it, and if you can afford it, go as organic as you can. If not, be sure to wash all produce very thoroughly to remove chemical residues.

Be conscious about your eating. When we use food to medicate pain, we tend to eat without being attentive to what we are actually putting into our bodies and what impact that food will have. Self-sabotaging behavior is a common thing in people who have been traumatized, and eating lots of junk is one of the most common self-sabotaging behaviors I have seen in trauma survivors.

Begin to pay attention to what you eat. For some, a food journal can help with this: write down what you eat and how you are feeling before, during, and after eating it. This can have dramatic effect, without your even trying to alter anything about your behavior. Once you become aware of the relationship between eating habits and emotions, it's hard to go on eating garbage.

Avoid problem foods. There are certain foods that people of African descent should avoid altogether. As an African-American myself, I've experienced firsthand how these foods disagree with me, and I've seen it in a lot of others. I've also seen how adhering to a diet that is as close as possible to the diets of my ancestors back in Africa has the most salutary effect on my physical well-being.

I'm not talking about hard-core science here; I'm talking about the education you can only get from trying something and seeing how much better it makes you feel.

Beyond the notion of eating right for your blood type, there are certain foods that tend to disagree with African-Americans that are embraced as healthy and necessary by the American mainstream. African-Americans are more likely to be lactose intolerant than whites. This means that they are missing an enzyme called lactase, which is needed in the digestive system to break down the sugar molecules (lactose) found in milk and milk products. When we eat dairy, the lactose goes through us undigested, and this causes gas, cramping, and diarrhea as it finds its way out.

The nutritional experts tell us that we need milk for its calcium, that African-Americans are at greater risk for cardiovascular disease and colon cancer because we don't consume enough dairy. The fine print of many of these studies shows us that they are funded by the dairy industry. Conflict of interest? You bet!

Babies should only drink milk from their mothers. Breastfeeding can go on until a child is one or even two years old—the World Health Organization recommends at least one full year. After they are weaned from the breast, there's no reason children need to drink milk, or eat macaroni and cheese.

It is true that if lactose intolerant people really want to eat dairy, they can learn to tolerate it better by eating it every day. One dairy food that seems exceptionally healthy is yogurt. Research has shown us that cultures that eat lots of yogurt have lower incidences of chronic disease and live longer lives.

I'm not talking about the kind of yogurt that's full of sugar and artificial flavorings; I'm talking about the plain kind, that has a bit of sourness to it, that's made with those healthy probiotic bacteria. The friendly bacteria added to the yogurt actually break down most of the lactose, and the bacteria go into your colon and help you to digest other foods and assimilate their nutrients. Plain yogurt can be sweetened with a little maple syrup or preserves, or with cut-up fresh fruit.

Wheat is in practically every processed food you find on supermarket shelves. Unfortunately, it also poses a problem for many African-Americans. Many of us have a hard time digesting it; others of us have subtle allergic reactions to it. Wheat allergy isn't well-recognized by the medical establishment, but keep in mind that wheat wasn't used in biblical times. It's a relatively new addition to the human diet, and we've gone from not having it at all to having it at practically every meal and snack. Many of us make antibodies in response to the proteins in wheat, and we end up with allergies and eczema and mood swings due to a subtle state of allergic inflammation in the body.

African-Americans would do well to eat a lot less wheat. Spelt, millet, quinoa, rice, corn, and chickpeas can be used instead, eaten as whole grains or used as flour.

Broccoli, cauliflower, and cabbage are widely recommended, and these are very healthy foods for some; but in others, the gastrointestinal distress they cause is a good indication that our bodies weren't made to eat them. Leafy greens are every bit as nutritious and easier for us to digest: collard and mustard greens, chard, kale, spinach, lettuces, baby greens, arugula.

That's it, in a nutshell. Eat foods the way the Creator made them; cultivate awareness about what and why you eat; and avoid problem foods. You don't need to count calories if you follow these guidelines, and you can "cheat" once in a while, but if you follow these guidelines overall you will be healthier and leaner in a matter of months.

Everyone will benefit from taking a good multivitamin. Go to a health food store and buy a high-potency multivitamin made from whole food ingredients. Those who don't like to swallow pills can take liquid versions. Women should take extra calcium/magnesium/vitamin D for bone health (1000 mg/500 mg/100 IU) every day.

Fasting and Purification

Fasting has long been a part of spiritual cleansing. Most major religions include periods of fasting. Consider fasting for yourself if you don't already do it as part of your religious practices. A two—to five-day fast can do amazing things for your body, cleansing it of toxins. Fasting also helps you to break unhealthy eating patterns and destructive relationships with food.

Go without food for five days? You have got to be joking. Most of us can go for weeks without food, and all that will happen is we'll lose a bunch of weight. After the first day or two of feeling hungry, the sensation stops. I've fasted many times and after the first two days, I don't even want food.

If you want to try fasting, make sure you eat only wholesome foods in the days before starting. Drink plenty of water and teas throughout the fast. When it comes time to break the fast, do so gently, starting with cooked grains, fruit, and vegetables and slowly working back into your normal diet.

Anyone who has a chronic medical condition, who takes medications, or who is pregnant or nursing a baby should avoid complete fasting. Instead, try a fruit and vegetable fast: eat only cooked vegetables, greens, and fruit for a few days. An enema each morning will help to move the cleansing process along, or try finding a colon hydrotherapist who you can visit for a high colonic. This is especially a good idea for those who eat a lot of meat. Meat digests slowly and can cause putrefaction in the colon. You need to go in there and cleanse it out periodically. Don't take any vitamins or herbs during a fast.

Women who have cellulite will find that fasting is the best way to dissolve it away. That dimpled appearance is from toxicity that flushes away when you fast.

Get Fit, Stay Fit

Exercise is usually the first thing to go when we get busy or stressed. For many of us, it was never even on the radar. Many of the nation's celebrity athletes are African-American; hip-hop dance is hugely popular, and the world has African-Americans to thank for creating this awesome dance form. In short, we have some great role models when it comes to working our bodies. Far too many of us fail to do so, however, at least on a regular basis. Too many of us sit on the couch and *watch* our black brothers and sisters play sports and dance on television, but have no desire to do the same.

Modern life puts the television and the computer higher on our lists of things to do than keeping fit. Inner-city residents have a slightly easier time staying active than those who live in the suburbs, because they still have to walk to get places. The fattest places in America are the suburbs. To get anywhere, suburbanites have to get in their cars.

A lot of the problem has to do with depression. Those who sit on the couch and eat and live their lives through soap operas and talk shows are doing so because they are depressed. They don't want to think, don't want to feel, don't want to take any risks. When talk-show hosts exhort them to get up off the couch and get some exercise, they might do so, but the irony is easy to see: they're being told to be active by the person they make a point of sitting on the couch to watch!

I made the point earlier in this chapter that we have to think of ourselves as worth the time and expense it takes to eat healthy. I feel the same way about exercise. Personally, I like Pilates the best. I go to a gym to use the Pilates equipment, and I feel strong and secure in my body and I am at a very healthy weight. I do cardiovascular exercise, too. Yes, Pilates is costly, but I think I'm worth it.

Whether you like basketball, hip-hop, yoga, or aerobics classes, get yourself into a program that includes both strengthening exercise (where you lift weights or your own body weight to strengthen muscles) and cardiovascular exercise. Stretching is a good idea, too, and this is one reason why I like Pilates so much—you work through the whole range of motion, so that you build strength and muscle length at the same time. Pilates also works the core muscles in the trunk, so that the back stays strong and you're resistant to back pain and injury. Yoga does many of the same things for you: it stretches and strengthens. Both yoga and Pilates involved focused breathing. Yoga students learn a bit more about relaxation and meditation—excellent for traumatized, stressed people.

Exercise should be part of every day. Cleaning your house, taking a walk, or anything else that keeps you moving and on your feet will help keep you fit, but engage in some kind of focused physical activity at least three times a week.

Herbs and Bach Flower Essences

In addition to my training as a psychologist, I've been studying herbology for some time now. One of my favorite natural remedies is the Bach flower essences. These are homeopathic remedies that work on Dr. Bach's statement that "health depends on being in harmony with our souls." Instead of masking conditions and symptoms with medications, these essences go to the root and treat the cause.

I recommend that women carry the Bach rescue remedy in their purses. It's wonderful for defusing stress and bringing relaxation. At this writing, I'm working on my own flower essence, which I hope to add to Dr. Bach's 38 other flower essences and those that have been developed by modern scientists.

Homeopaths and naturopaths can prescribe flower essences for you. They may seem unfounded in hard science, but they really work.

Herbs, on the other hand, are gaining a lot of scientific attention. More and more people are using herbs to try to treat symptoms of illness. Herbs don't work that way, though—they are great for moving the body towards balance, but they don't work like "magic bullets" to target specific disease processes.

If you are interested in using herbs to counteract stress, try valerian, passionflower, or chamomile, as tinctures, teas, or capsules. If you want to use herbs to energize your body and mind, you can try Siberian ginseng or other ginsengs, or ginkgo biloba. A good reference on herbs and vitamins for achieving physical and mental balance is Earl Mindell, RPh, PhD's book, *Prescription Alternatives* (written with Virginia Hopkins, M.A.; McGraw Hill, 2003).

Chapter Eight

Calling the Clan Together

The impersonal hand of government can never replace the helping hand of a neighbor.

—Hubert H. Humphrey, address in Washington, D.C., February 10, 1965.

I have fond memories of my childhood in Philadelphia. I lived in a tightly knit community, where everyone knew everyone else. All the kids in my neighborhood knew one another and we played with the neighborhood children almost as much as we did with siblings. Our mothers almost all were home to watch over us, but they allowed us a lot of freedom to play and roam as long as we were good boys and girls. We all felt protected and watched over. No one worried about being cut down by a stray bullet, or being attacked or raped. We felt safe. Our grandparents were around, and so were our aunts and uncles and cousins. In the humid summer evenings, everyone would sit outside, talking and laughing and eating.

That was our clan. That was the soil from which I grew to be what I am today.

In every town, in every village, every city, every suburb, things have changed. The people sit inside their houses and apartments—which, in many cases, might be bumped right up next to one another, or very close to one another—and watch TV and eat and sleep and surf the Internet, with virtually no contact with anyone outside of their immediate household unit. When they go out, they hop into their cars and zoom away to school or work. Perhaps they manage a "hello" for a neighbor before dialing someone on their cell phones or tuning into a morning radio show.

People feel far less attached to where they live, and move from place to place with unprecedented ease. People live, work, attend school, and recreate in places that are far apart from one another. There is very little attachment to community, in both geographic and social realms.

Sure, we have friendships, and many of us have strong connections through church and our children's schools and other activities. But we have lost that unique combination of geographic proximity and cooperative, supportive, attentive individuals that brings about the kind of safety most of us can't even imagine anymore—the kind of community that lifts and supports each individual and pushes them to be and do their best.

Human beings evolved not as individuals, but as communities. Despite Western conceptualizations, the smallest functional unit of humankind is not the individual—it is the clan. No individual, no single parent-child dyad, no nuclear family could survive alone. We survived and evolved as clans—interdependent—socially, emotionally and biologically. Children belong to the community; they are entrusted to parents.

—Bruce Perry

In some parts of some cities, African-American clanship is still alive and kicking, with one significant difference: most of the mothers work outside of the home. Children go unsupervised for too much of the time, and they get into trouble. They start to seek out the kind of strong community that they know they lack.

They start to look for safety. They long to feel like someone is watching their backs. In a world that seems geared to defeat any hopes or ambitions these children have, the search for ways to get ahead in the world in terms of financial and social status begins early. This is how children end up involved in gangs.

Gangs Are Not New

African-American gangs have been around since the 1920s. In their beginnings, these gangs were rarely involved in violence, or even in territorial disputes; they consisted of members of a clan—family members, neighbors—who would engage in some sort of criminal behavior. Early gang members were out to establish their place in the social hierarchy or to earn money without backbreaking work.

In those days, there was fighting between rival gangs, but there were rules about how to fight. If you didn't fight fair, you were ostracized. Gangs might have done crimes, but they were also places where young people could feel that they were part of a tribe without also being in mortal danger at every turn. Today, everyone has a gun, and merely wearing the wrong color or flashing the wrong hand sign can get you killed in some parts of America, and fighting fair isn't part of the game anymore.

By 1960, South Central LA and Compton were home to the main African-American gangs. The Crips and the Bloods—the best-known and most feared of these gangs—began to take over neighborhoods and commit strong-arm robberies in the latter part of that decade. Their tactics became increasingly vicious. Both the Crips and the Bloods divided into smaller gangs ("sets") in the 1970s, and gang warfare began in earnest around that time. By the 1980s, the number of Crips and Bloods in the LA area reached about 15,000, with the typical gang member aged 14 to 24.

The criminal activities of gangs include drug trafficking (mainly marijuana, crack, PCP, and LSD), burglary, robbery, and assault. Gang activity in prisons is intense; many young African-Americans join gangs for the first time while in prison.

By far, the worst problem with gangs today is that they do a lot of killing. Between January and November of 2002, 583 homicides were committed in the Los Angeles area. This number was as high as the total homicides in LA for the entire year of 2001. In one four-day period, there were 13 murders committed in this second-largest city in the U.S. It is not known how many of these hundreds of murders were gang-related, but it is likely that the majority of them were.

Reports of drive-by shootings and other gang-related homicides or attempted homicides can be found almost daily in the *LA Times*. Many of those who die at the hands of gang members are children: children who got in the way of a stray bullet, or who were otherwise in the wrong place at the wrong time.

In one incident, 13-year-old Quinesha Dunford and 13-year-old Demario Moore, students at an LA arts high school, were standing in front of an alleyway in South Los Angeles at around 7:00 in the evening. They were shot from a passing car. Quinesha died after making her way to a nearby house; Demario died in an ambulance. A bystander caught a glimpse of the license plate number of the car, and an 18-year-old, a 16-year-old, and a 17-year-old were arrested for the killings. The police reported that the killings had to do with a long-standing conflict between two rival gangs, but that the kids who had been killed had no gang affiliation.

More recently, two boys who lived in LA were pressured by gang members to reveal their gang affiliation. The boys refused, because they had made a point of not joining any gang. They were killed for their refusal.

Hundreds more stories like this are begging to be told. No matter how the details go, those of us who have never been part of a gang have the same response: we wonder how on earth this could be happening. How could children do this to other children?

If you wonder how a fourteen-year-old can shoot another child his own age in the head, or how boys can do "drive-by shootings" and then go home to dinner, you need to know you don't get there in a day, or week, or month. It takes years of preparation to be willing to commit murder, to be willing to kill or die for a corner, a color, or a leather jacket…

While killing another person is not natural, it's not that difficult to learn… Wars abound—intentional starvation, the killing of civilians, women and children—and these atrocities are sometimes committed by farmers, laborers, and other ordinary people. Even in this country, the military can take an eighteen-year-old boy and turn him into a killer in a matter of months. People can be taught *to kill. And children growing up under the conditions of war that we find in many poor communities today learn to think about death and killing as a matter of survival. And of course there are always those who are willing to teach children how to kill, and how to die.*

These are usually the real role models in our inner cities, older boys and girls who teach the codes of conduct and enforce the rules of order.

—Geoffrey Canada, *FistStickKnifeGun: A Personal History of Violence in America,* Beacon Press, Boston, MA, 1995: p. 35-36.

Children who join gangs learn how to do violence and how to kill. Violence and killing—along with money, made through the trafficking of illegal drugs—are the currency that is dealt amongst these young people. To be accepted into a gang, most have to go through a sort of hazing where they fight someone within the gang, commit a crime, or initiate violence against a rival gang. Daily exposure to violent power struggles numbs these children to the emotional impact of that violence.

They are willing to undergo the transformation from child to gang member because they are in need of a clan. This particular clan happens to indoctrinate them into a way of life that is steeped in violence. In return for their devotion and loyalty, these children experience a deep familial love and support that they may not have gotten from their family of origin.

Gang Culture: The Urban Tribe

African-American gangs were, originally, a tribe within a tribe. They existed secondary to the larger clan of African-American families. As the family deteriorated, the gangs took on greater significance. Eventually, gang life became a replacement for family and neighborhood life that had become fractured beyond recognition. Children didn't get the support they needed to deal with traumas, and so they began to turn to gangs for that support. Sadly, gang life creates terrifying trauma even as it supports its members' getting through it. This duality only increases the strength of the bonds between gang members.

Modern urban street gangs have evolved into tribal organizational structures. These new urban tribes have developed into a subculture in the streets of the urban jungle. They claim territory, are self-supporting, have their own language and customs, and establish their own rules and codes of conduct. Their customs are passed to new members by rites of passage from generation to generation, thus ensuring the continuance of the gang. Gang members identify themselves as a people that is separate from the rest of society.

—Mike Carlie, Ph.D., "Into the Abyss: A Personal Journey into the World of Street Gangs," after Etter, 1999: p. 261.

When I refer to the tribe or to the clan, I'm really talking about *society.* A society is a social group that endures and cooperates through organized relationships with one another; it embraces a culture, which Schaefer defines as "the totality of learned, socially transmitted customs, knowledge, material objects, and behavior." Human beings need society; many animal species have societies, too, but they don't have culture. Culture is distinctly human.

If you rob human beings of either, they will create it anew. This is what has happened with gangs in the inner cities. The feeling of belonging, of being needed, of walking into the fire with someone watching your back is far more alluring to young, poor African-Americans than anything else anyone is offering them right now.

Children need connectedness and strong social support to deal with and move past trauma. If we are to save our children from gang life, we must make it less attractive; and the only way to do that is to strengthen the tribe that consists of parents, aunts, uncles, cousins, neighborhood, community, church, and society. We must provide culture and strong emotional and practical support, sisterhood and brotherhood, and places of worship where children feel taken care of.

Bringing Back the Safety of Human Touch

Human nature is such that every person needs to feel important. In our first weeks, months, and years on this earth, the kind of attention we receive from our parents and from our clan establishes whether we feel important or unimportant. The message we get in early life is going to have a lot to do with how we esteem ourselves in the years to come. The language with which this is communicated to the clan's youngest members is touch.

From the time a baby is born, it needs to be touched, held, caressed, and hugged. Even before giving birth, mothers instinctively caress their growing bellies, and the baby inside feels and responds to this. Without this kind of stimulation, the nervous system doesn't develop properly, and children come to believe that their needs are not going to be met in this life.

There is no human being that does not respond to touch. We can move people from irrational to rational just by touching them.

I, for one, have begun to recoil against human touch, and so have a lot of other people. I'll tell you why: it's because something that is meant to be safe has been made unsafe. The powerful instincts towards nestling together, holding one another, and caressing one another are being countered by an undercurrent of fear. Children as young as preschool age are warned about "inappropriate touching," and as adults, we are afraid to touch children in the way they need to be touched, for fear of being inappropriate.

The culture at large has begun to sexualize virtually everything, including the innocent and necessary touching that goes on within immediate family and within the clan. This is tragic.

How do we get back to the safety we need in order to be comfortable with touch again? It's the clan that brings us to that safety. It is with the familiarity of the mother's touch, the father's touch, the touch of siblings that we begin to feel that touching is safe. The nuclear family is the basis of the larger clan, the smallest functional unit.

A new mother with her baby instinctively touches and caresses the child. She kisses her, nibbles her toes, wiggles her hands and feet, rocks and bounces her. Many times, I've seen a new mother who has handed her baby off to someone else continuing to bounce and rock and rub her own arms as though she were still holding the child. It's ingrained into us to act this way, and it serves an important purpose.

The mother's touch is never as tender or nurturing as when a baby feeds at the breast. Only about 68 percent of new mothers even attempt to breastfeed their babies, and by the six-month mark, only 31 percent are still breastfeeding. (The World Health Organization and the American Academy of Pediatrics recommend that all babies nurse for at least one year, and that they get breast milk exclusively for the first six months.) It is possible to bottle-feed tenderly and with lots of touching, but often the convenience of sticking a bottle in the mouth of a baby while it's in a car seat or some other kind of child-holding contraption wins out. Bottle-feeding can be done by anyone, anywhere, and the loss of that intimate skin-to-skin touching and nourishment hurts clan-building (and self-esteem) at its deepest roots.

Today, there are all sorts of contraptions—strollers, playpens, bouncers, electronically powered swings, walkers, "interactive" toys—designed to provide stimulation and movement for babies. We've been duped into believing that these things will improve the intelligence and motor skills of babies, that they are perfectly good substitutes for the loving and responsive touch and time of a caring adult or older child. *They are not.* If you raise a child with these kinds of objects, don't be surprised when they care more about material things than people.

A father's touch is not as tender as a mother's, but it's safe. The father throws the child up in the air, playing, laughing, risking—but he always catches the child when he falls back towards the ground. From this kind of play, we learn trust; we learn that risk and a little edge of fear doesn't mean that we are not safe. Someone is watching our backs.

We need to remove the touch of Cain and Abel, and bring the good sibling touch back. In this day, siblings tend to be competitive rather than cooperative. When they are being raised by a single parent without the support of the clan, this competition can become intense. The context of the tribe brings an openness to the nuclear family,. This gives giving siblings more freedom to interact with children of other parents and with adults other than the parents,. They no longer need to removing the feeling that they must fight tooth and nail for attention from the same adult.

Honoring our Elders

When we call the clan together, we have to honor the elders. This is what will make them want to stick around. In American culture, youth and sexual attractiveness are valued above the experience and wisdom of age. Elders are not given the respect they deserve. It's no wonder they don't want to remain a part of the clan.

The current trend towards elderly people living together in "senior living" communities is deadly for the life of the tribe. Clans are intergenerational, and they need elders more now than they ever have—but many elders are choosing instead to remove themselves from the community and enter one made up of people their own age. While this kind of life might be easier because it disengages elders from certain kinds of troubles, it robs them of feeling needed, and it robs the clan of the wisdom of age.

Instead of going to be with the grandparents or the aunt or uncle when Mom is at work, children go to day-care centers staffed by underpaid workers, where they are not touched and where they do not feel important.

Humans instinctively create social hierarchies within clans. As long as we remember to respect our elders, the rest of the hierarchy falls into place. We must remember to give our elders first right to be spokespersons within the clan, to respect them as holders of wisdom—not to look down upon them because they're not "with the times" or because they don't look like a picture from a fashion magazine!

Making Space for Children to be Children

When a clan of elephants is under threat, they gather in a circle with the babies in the center. We need to do this for our own children. The clan protects children against that which they are not developmentally able to handle. This includes inappropriate sexual stimuli and exposure to violence.

Let's not forget that many of the sexual and violent acts visited upon young children come from within families, within networks of family friends and acquaintances. But if our tribes were cohesive, if we were really keeping track of one another, no man would dare mess with women or children. The consequences would be far too dire. Jail time and the other threats of the criminal justice system pale in comparison to being shunned by the clan that you have been a part of since you were born.

The clan gives children the strength to resist drugs and premarital sex, because it gives children the feeling that what they do in their lives is too important to throw away through addiction or premature motherhood—and not only to themselves.

Reinforcing appropriate dietary choices is another role of the clan. It applies constructive social pressure and direct guidance to children, showing them the way through example.

The beleaguered public school system has been left holding the bag on a good many of the problems that should be handled by the tribe. Schools are expected to teach kids about sexuality, nutrition, and drugs. They are expected to deal with violence (and sex) between children that has reached a scale never before witnessed in civilized society. Teachers, administrators, curriculum designers, and school counselors struggle to keep kids on track, but doing so is virtually impossible without the support of children's families. Without the support of the clan, families can't do it all, either. Everyone loses.

Mentorship programs also seek to fill the void where the tribe should be. Those who choose to mentor are doing a wonderful thing, but this is passing the buck. When a parents allows a mentor to take on a significant role in their child's life, they are giving away responsibility. They are giving away ownership of their child's present and future.

By the time a child gets to school, they should already be prepared to learn, to receive the gift of education. The most malleable state of a child's brain exists during the preschool years; by the time they enter kindergarten, their path is pretty much established. Establishing the early groundwork of the child's path to a successful life isn't the job of anyone but the parents and their clan. We need to turn off TV and spend time with our young children reading and exploring and appreciating the wonders of science, literature, mathematics, history, writing, art. This is not an easy thing to do when our parents did not do so for us, but if we are to break the cycle of violence and trauma, it has to be done.

The Church and the Clan

For many African-Americans, the church is where their clan is. The pastor or priest or minister is their guide. Unfortunately, pastors and other religious leaders are failing to take a strong enough role in forming and maintaining clans within the African-American community.

Most churches raise funds through tithing. In poor areas, many of those who give money every Sunday when the hat is passed are living below the poverty line. I have seen elders whose electricity has been shut off for lack of payment, giving money to their churches. This is wrong. Churches should be giving more than they take. Once they have done the job of empowering their parishoners, *then* they can think about tithing.

If any one group of people can reinvent the clan, it is our religious and spiritual leaders. They are the ones who held us together in slave days, and we need them to help us to revisit that clanship without the burden of slavery.

Intentional Community: The Modern Clan

Wouldn't it be nice if our families could stick together? If the generations could stay within a specific geographical area, preferably the same neighborhood? That might just solve a lot of problems. If children didn't move out of state when they grew up…if elders didn't head off to old folks' homes…if parents didn't split up and move hundreds of miles apart…if economic concerns didn't move families apart…if, if, if.

Okay, so, if this isn't possible, how do we move back into community? In today's world, where geographical borders are blurred and where the search for opportunity and adventure take us far from our places of birth, we have to change the definition of the clan. We have to move it into the 21st century. It has to take on the fluidity that modern life has developed due to both real and virtual access to many worlds outside of the one in which we were raised.

To rebuild American community, we must approach the task with *intention.* We must look at the end result we desire, and work from there. Too many of us have forgotten *how* to be part of a clan. That spirit of selflessness, cooperation, compassion, and collectivity has all but disappeared these days; it's every man, woman, and child for themselves.

Unless we *intend* to live in community with others, it is too easy to reject the difficult aspects and so reject the whole notion. Creating community requires cooperation; it requires time and effort spent ironing things out with like-minded (and, sometimes, not-so-like-minded) people. It requires a skilled approach to the resolution of conflict. Each member must make a contribution. At times, it may seem easier to give up and go back into our darkened living rooms, remote at the ready.

Modern communes, kibbutzes, other types of religious, spiritual, and secular designed communities, some group houses, communities designed around sustainable and energy-efficient living, "back-to-the-land" groups that live rurally, and housing cooperatives are all examples of *intentional community.*

Like fish who always swim out of water and therefore remain unaware of it, we live in a toxic fog of frustrating living situations. They do not nurture us, they do not encourage our natural cooperative sides, they are not even fun on a day-by-day basis, and they keep us from the awareness that it isn't necessary to live this way. All they do is keep up our standing as credit-card-carrying consumer-zombies. But life is more than working and buying, and we need a built environment that will encourage more than commercial interactions among us...

What is needed is to re-create the virtues we crave in small towns—their personal intimacy, their sense of mutual support (and forbearance), their slower personal pace, their feeling of a shared community destiny—but do it everywhere, in cities and urban suburbs where most of us in fact live.

—Ernest Callenbach, foreword to Ken Norwood, AICP and Kathleen Smith's *Rebuilding Community in America: Housing for Ecological Living, Personal Empowerment, and the New Extended Family,* Shared Living Resource Center, Berkeley, CA:1995.

Intentional community consists of a group of people who make the choice to live as a clan. Hundreds of these kinds of communities exist all over the world, in a variety of forms. Some are built from the ground up, complete with individual dwellings, group gathering space, workshop space, community gardens, playgrounds, and open space. Others are created in apartment complexes or houses in the inner city, rurally, or in suburbs.

There are many ways to go about creating community. The major challenges are gathering people together who are interested enough to make it happen; and to raise the needed funds for this kind of venture.

Types of Intentional Community

All of these types of housing have the advantages of bringing people together. Those who live in intentional communities are able to share responsibilities so that they have more free time.

Commune: a group of individuals who share land and other assets and who share income and resources with one another. Kibbutzim are Israeli communal living arrangements.

Cohousing: short for "cooperative housing;" describes a kind of housing ownership where those who live in the housing create a corporation that owns that housing. The members of the housing co-op own shares of that co-op. There are many versions of cooperative housing, depending upon the needs of the members and the climate of the housing market.

Condominium: yes, condos are a kind of intentional community. Each unit is privately owned and there is shared common space. A board makes decisions about management and operation, and each condominium owner is responsible for following rules pertaining to common areas.

Eco-village: an intentional community that emphasizes environmental preservation, sustainability, and the growth of community gardens. These communities promote health and well-being by going back to nature: there is little reliance on cars or fossil fuels, and more emphasis on public transportation and alternative transportation and energy sources. Eco-villages have non-profit forms of ownership of land and housing.

Group Home: a home that serves those who have special needs, such as teenaged mothers, recovering alcoholics or drug addicts, elderly, disabled, or young wards of the court.

Spiritual Community: any intentional community that centers around a shared religious or spiritual belief.

Urban Cooperative Block: where groups of urban dwellers agree to create common space by knocking down backyard fences. Gardens, hot tubs, new buildings for group use, and play space for children can be created in the new open space.

Group House: Usually a group of unrelated individuals who share a single commonly owned or rented dwelling. Meals and chores are shared, as are the common spaces in the house.

Intergenerational community: unfortunately, many existing intentional communities do not welcome children or elderly people. Intergenerational communities are specifically designed to include people of all ages.

Definitions from Rebuilding Community in America by Ken Norwood, AICP, and Kathleen Smith

The purposes of intentional communities vary. Some "have been formed to share resources, to create great family neighborhoods, to live ecologically sustainable lifestyles, or to live with others who hold similar values. Some communities are wholly secular; others are committed to a common spiritual practice; many are spiritually eclectic. Some are focused on egalitarian values and voluntary simplicity, or mutual interpersonal growth work, or rural homesteading and self-reliance. Some communities provide services, for example helping war refugees, the urban homeless, or developmentally disabled children or adults. Some communities operate rural conference and retreat centers, health and healing centers, or sustainable-living education centers." (From the Intentional Community Web Site, www.ic.org/.)

If you are interested in exploring intentional communities—either for the purpose of starting one or of joining one that has already been established—here are a few ways you can begin. Contact:

The Intentional Community Web Site, at www.ic.org/

The Cohousing Association of America, at www.cohousing.org/

The Foundation for Community Encouragement, at www.fce-community.org

This website was founded by Scott Peck, a Christian psychiatrist. If you are interested in trying to create community without changing your living situation, this website is a good resource for you.

The Shared Living Resource Center, at www.sharedliving.org/

This is where you can purchase the book quoted above, Rebuilding Community in America*—a great resource for anyone who is serious about wanting to live in an intentional community.*

You don't have to pack up your kids and move into a commune to benefit from intentional community. Simply holding the intention of creating community in your mind and heart may be all you need to do. This will foster your desire to connect with others and to strengthen your ties to the community in which you already live.

Start With A Community Garden

Ancient clans developed around food sources. People would settle where food and water were plentiful. Today's clans can do the same, although food is now available just about everywhere. In cities where urban gardens are planted, this is happening right now.

Urban gardens are plots of land upon which a group of people does the work of cultivating fruits, vegetables, and flowers. They are collective efforts, shared by communities, and the harvest from those gardens are also shared. It's a beautiful thing to see inner-city children dig their hands into soil for the first time; to see them gobble down green vegetables that taste wonderful to them because they watched them grow from a seedling.

In Koshland Park, San Fransisco, Barbara Wenger gathered the efforts of local high school students and residents of two urban housing projects to develop and tend an urban garden. On a corner that had once been ruled by drugs and prostitution, there arose a lush garden. In Newark, New Jersey, the Reverend Anna Holder created a 17-plot garden within a mostly African-American and

Latino community. In 1992, right after the L.A. riots, teachers at Crenshaw High School started a garden that eventually gave rise to Food from the 'Hood, a student-run business that sells Straight Out 'the Garden salad dressing to major supermarket chains. The garden is a teaching laboratory for kids in the inner city—it teaches agriculture and entrepreneurship—and yields wholesome foods for community members.

Since the 1970s, over 550 community gardens have sprung up around the nation. The American Community Gardening Association (ACGA) lends support and instruction to those who wish to follow suit.

You can reach them at www.communitygarden.org/.

Chapter Nine

Cognitive Psychology, Cognitive Therapy; Or, Therapy Isn't Just For White People

Much of the "counseling" that goes on in the African-American community goes on at the kitchen table—that warm, inviting, comfortable place, filled with the smells and sounds of home. Mothers and daughters, fathers and sons, sisters and brothers, cousins, friends sit down at the kitchen table and talk about their lives and try to support one another the best they know how.

I don't wish to minimize the importance of this kind of therapy. It is at the core of the clan, and it is a part of the glue that holds communities and families together. In one of my satellite offices in Philadelphia, I even created a kitchen environment where therapists and patients could interact more comfortably. But a lot of African-Americans believe that the kitchen table is their version of therapy—that it is every bit as helpful, or more so, compared with the therapy administered by trained professional therapists. This belief is incorrect, and it keeps a lot of traumatized, damaged people out of therapy.

At the kitchen table, at the barbershops, at the hair salons, we feel warm and fuzzy and loved and embraced, but we have failed to get to the root of problems. We have not broken looming silences or aired necessary truths. We bandage the wounds instead of cleaning them out and letting them be exposed to the light of day so that they can finally and completely heal.

Perhaps in the old days, when our lives were simpler and our communities more cohesive, when our expectations of ourselves and others were a part of an unwritten code that everyone understood, kitchen-table counseling *was* all we needed. But today, as we continue to be caught up in cycles of violence and trauma and hatred, we need a reality check. We need to re-learn how to think and behave in peaceful ways. We need to find our own strength and to allow that strength to carry us through whatever traumas we must face. And we can't do that at the kitchen table anymore.

There's a saying that was popularized by the 12-step group Alcoholics Anonymous: *Insanity is doing the same thing over and over and expecting the results to be different.* We keep going back to the kitchen table, and we keep losing our children to violence. Something has to be done differently.

Throughout this book, I have tried to make it clear that therapists alone cannot heal the aftermath of trauma. We need community, we need holistic healing, we need clergy, we need to raise our children in a new way. But there is a place for therapy in this picture of healing, and it cannot be left out in most instances. Rarely, individuals have the wherewithal and the self-knowledge and the insight to move through trauma and stay healthy. Those of us who aren't able to do this should not feel badly; it is a rare thing indeed.

On the other hand, let me be clear that African-Americans' aversion to therapist-delivered psychotherapy is not unfounded. At the kitchen table, we feel accepted, we feel that our cultural heritage is being honored; this is often not the case on the therapist's couch.

The systems that have been created to help the less privileged to get into therapy are not exactly user-friendly. Paperwork and other bureaucratic nonsense is enough to deter many of those who go into the system to try to get the help they need, and those who plunge into that fray often end up being retraumatized by insensitive therapists and institutions who don't understand where they're coming from.

In the not-so-distant past, blacks were far more likely to be institutionalized, misdiagnosed, surgically altered, or treated with dangerous drugs when they sought help for mental illness. Not so long ago, blacks who were deemed to be mentally infirm were among those that were sterilized against their will.

Today's typical therapeutic environment is based on mainstream America, and this hasn't worked for African-Americans. There has been little cultural sensitivity in psychotherapists' offices, and this needs to change if we as therapists are to help those most vulnerable to trauma—blacks, Latinos, and Asians, all of whom are falling into the abyss of gang violence on an ever-increasing scale.

A few of my colleagues were treating a young Asian woman who periodically would exhibit symptoms similar to those of paranoid schizophrenia. She was on the verge of being committed to an institution. Fortunately, one of us realized that her problem was not psychological, but cultural.

In Asian families, the youngest child is responsible for the elder of the family. Every time therapists talked to this woman—who happened to be the youngest child in her family—about some aspect of treatment that would separate her from this elder, her paranoid symptoms would come up. The therapists' lack of understanding of her culture was causing them both to misdiagnose and retraumatize her.

Therapy That Works

What comes to your mind when you hear the word *psychotherapy*? Do you picture a well-dressed, upper-middle-class white person lying on a couch and staring into space, talking to a well-dressed, upper-middle-class white person sitting in a chair with a notepad? Or do you picture a bunch of raggedy, distressed-looking folks sitting in a circle, drinking coffee and being guided through a group therapy session? Something in between?

Since its earliest manifestations, psychotherapy has evolved into a number of methods and systems that are as different from one another as night is from day. There are many schools of thought about how best to help those who suffer from mental illness or who have difficulty coping with the demands their lives place upon them; some have proven more effective than others in clinical research.

Here are a few common misconceptions and truths held in the African-American community about psychotherapy:

MISCONCEPTION: *It usually takes at least a few years of therapy to heal from psychological problems.*

TRUTH: Actually, a good therapist should be able to heal a patient within a few months, with positive changes happening within a few weeks. Any therapist who keeps you as a patient for years and years isn't doing her job. Some patients get addicted to therapy, returning every week for years on end to have their hour, set aside exclusively for their whining and complaining. Any therapist that allows a patient to do this without guiding them towards solutions is also not doing his or her job.

MISCONCEPTION: *In therapy, the therapist's main job is to help the patient understand why his or her problems exist—for example, to get the patient to talk about his or her past traumas in a "safe" setting.*

TRUTH: It is true that some therapists focus almost exclusively on delving into the past. They do this because they believe that simply understanding the past will heal the patient in the present. This kind of "talk therapy" has a long history that started with Freud and his colleagues, and while it may help to bring up traumatic issues from the past—indeed, this is a necessary part of healing from trauma—there is more to therapy than this. More effective therapy techniques involve some looking backwards, but they focus strongly on the present and the future. Rather than talking about what is already impossible to change, therapy that works focuses on identifying and altering faulty, self-destructive ways of thinking and behaving, *today.*

MISCONCEPTION: *Therapy consists mostly of the patient talking and the therapist listening while asking a question now and then.*

TRUTH: Therapy that works should be like that class you took in college that you loved because you were interested, because there was lots of give-and-take, because you felt like you were really learning something valuable. A good therapist *teaches* you how to think and behave differently so that you can improve your life and your relationships. They'll even give you homework and check to make sure you've done it!

MISCONCEPTION: *Therapy is too expensive.*

TRUTH: If you have been wounded by trauma, or if you are depressed or anxious, if your relationships feel unsatisfying, you can't afford *not* to seek this kind of help. A good therapist can help you make big changes within five to 15 sessions—an investment that will enrich the remainder of your days on Earth. Many therapists will work with you to make payment plans, and many states have programs that enable low-income individuals and families to get therapeutic help. You might be able to get low-cost counseling from a student who is working towards a counseling degree.

These kinds of programs can be frustratingly inadequate; if you go into them knowing exactly what kind of therapy you want, you are much more likely to have a good experience.

You only go around once as the person you are in this life; don't let the cost of therapy stand between you and happiness. If you are in trouble, nothing else will be right if you don't fix it.

MISCONCEPTION: *If you have good friends, trusted family members, or trusted clergy to talk to about your problems, you don't need psychotherapy.*

See the beginning of this chapter. The kitchen table isn't cutting it anymore, and clergy don't have the training to help you change the way you think. Trauma has deep effects on *how you think,* and the changes that go on in your thinking have deep effects on your behavior that you might not even know about. It's practically impossible to see these things from inside yourself. You need a pair of eyes and a heart and a mind that are trained specifically to identify flawed thought patterns, and that are trained to teach you how to change them.

MISCONCEPTION: *People who go into therapy are weak. A person should be able to handle his own problems.*

TRUTH: On the contrary—being able to admit that you need therapy is a sign of great strength. Before a person agrees to therapy, he has to be able to admit that there is something in him that is broken, something that needs repairing. This in itself takes courage. For many African-Americans, this is the most difficult hurdle of all. Once they've managed to admit to themselves that they need to get some help, doing so—and healing—feels easy in comparison.

In this Q&A, I've been describing the kind of therapy I do in my own practice, and that I have found to be most effective for the treatment of just about every psychological problem that can be treated. It is called *cognitive-behavioral therapy.*

Cognitive-Behavioral Therapy: What To Expect

People's behaviors and feelings are strongly affected by the way in which they perceive the world. That perception is based on that person's unique history, his unique experience in this life. Flashing a gang sign might incite a traumatized gang member to rage (if it's a rival's sign) or feelings of brotherly love (if it's his own sign); flashing that same sign to a Fortune 500 CEO or a white Midwestern housewife will elicit little more than confusion.

Beneath those responses are what cognitive therapists call *automatic thoughts.* These are sometimes referred to as "self-talk," the internal monologue that goes on in our heads so often that we don't even realize it's there. Try this: the next time you feel depressed, anxious, or otherwise off-balance, stop and ask yourself: *What was going through my mind just then?* Start listening to those automatic thoughts. With the help of a good therapist, you will be able to see how those thoughts are holding you back.

Cognitive therapists help patients to take a cold, clear, dispassionate look at their core beliefs. Those beliefs shape our perception dramatically, causing us to focus on that which supports them and to pass by that which does not.

When a new patient begins therapy, the first thing I do is assess their present state of mind. I use assessment instruments that are modeled after those that have been created by mainstream psychology, but that have been altered to be more culturally sensitive. The assessment takes up the first two treatment sessions.

A Note on Culturally Competent Communication

In 1972, Robert L. Williams created the word "Ebonics" to describe the unique patois of African-Americans. Black children in newly integrated schools were already beginning to suffer because of a language barrier. Standardized tests didn't speak to these children. They weren't culturally relevant, and they weren't in a language that many African-American children felt at home speaking, reading, or writing.

The notion that African-American Vernacular English (AAVE), the linguists' name for black English, is somehow "slang" is a false one. It contains slang like any other language, and the popularity of hip-hop and rap music have cranked up the exposure of this slang to large numbers of impressionable young people. But AAVE is most definitely a *language,* with strict rules of word order and syntax, along with a distinctive lexicon: *homey, crib, phat, nigga, diss, wack, ashy, nappy.*

Young African-Americans are caught between pressures from integrated schools and institutions to speak the Queen's English and pressure from peers to speak in AAVE. Children who grow up in poor, inner-city, almost exclusively black neighborhoods enter school and struggle against what amounts to a language barrier. When they begin to speak in American English, they are told by their peers or family members, "You talk like a white boy" or "You talk like a white girl." Like many people who come from cultures where a different language is spoken, African-Americans often speak their vernacular in some situations and more "proper" English in others. Those who can consciously make the choice to do this are usually those who are in better socioeconomic straits; poor inner-city youth don't generally have that choice to make.

In a fascinating study by linguist William Labov, inner-city African-American children were given sentences to repeat back. They found it almost impossible to repeat the statements without making specific changes in word order:

Questioner: I asked Alvin if he could go.

Subject: I as' Alvin could he—could he go.

Questioner: I asked Alvin whether he knows how to play basketball.

Subject: I as' Alvin—I asked Alvin—I can't—I didn't quite hear you.

Questioner: I asked Alvin did he know how to play basketball.

Subject: I asked Alvin whether—did he know how to play basketball.

The linguistic patterns of AAVE are deep-seated, regular, governed by rules, and distinctive. Instead of "I don't know what that person is doing," it's "Ah on' know what homey be doin'." Instead of "She's had that handmade dress for a long time," it's "She BIN had dat han'made dress." Instead of "He has his thing, I have mine," it's "He got his thing, I got mine."

AAVE is what is known as a *creole*—a combination of more than one language. The AAVE spoken in New Orleans or in parts of Georgia—including Gullah, a dialect spoken by a shrinking group of Southern African-Americans—is different from the AAVE spoken in New York City.

Most Americans are at least somewhat familiar with AAVE constructions and slang terms because of the popularity of rap and hip-hop. But when it comes to book learning and school achievement and success in psychotherapy, AAVE creates barriers, and those barriers need to be addressed. I'm not suggesting that white therapists or teachers attempt to speak AAVE when dealing with African-Americans; this would most likely come off as insulting or comical. But they do need to *appreciate* this language and its roots in our cultural heritage. They need to have a rudimentary understanding of it.

Rather than regarding it as "lazy English" or nothing but street slang, we need to regard AAVE as a valid way of communicating—a way that is especially valuable for communicating the very experiences that make being African-American a potential source of trauma. In the *New Republic* (March 28, 1981), Toni Morrisson tells an interviewer that "there are certain things I cannot say without recourse to my [AAVE] language…I know the standard English. I want to use it to restore the other language, the *lingua franca.*"

In therapy, African-Americans who speak AAVE struggle to make themselves understood and to understand what the therapist is trying to teach them. The frustration of doing so can drive black people out of therapy. If we are to successfully deal with the problem of trauma in the African-American community, the therapeutic community must not only be knowledgeable about African-American culture, but must also understand and respect black English.

In the late 1990s, Oakland, California school board member Toni Cook proposed that the failure of African-American children to achieve in school could be remedied by teaching them in Ebonics. (This word was developed in the 1970s, a combination of "ebony" and "phonics" that was believed to sound better than "black English.") Her proposal raised a huge controversy, but its roots were sound: you can't teach children in a language they don't know. Cook, an African-American woman of great intelligence and eloquence, was labeled a racist. Ebonics became a polarizing factor in the continuing affirmative-action debate.

Today, Ebonics is taught in many colleges, and many of its distinctive words and phrases have entered into general usage. We must be careful, however, to preserve the original impact and unique expressiveness of the language as parts of it are mainstreamed.

Once I have a strong grasp of the patient's issues, I carefully create a treatment plan. The plan includes both short-term and long-term goals. I sit down with the patient and explain my basic findings, and spell out the goals I believe they can reach. Small goals, when consistently attained, are the stuff recovery is made of.

One woman I treated was a crack addict. Many of her teeth were missing, and at the beginning of therapy, she was an all-around mess. As we began to set goals for her recovery, she'd show up at each session a little neater, a little cleaner. She seemed to be inspired by my own groomed appearance. Lipstick and makeup didn't do much to improve her smile, however, because of the missing teeth. If I had brought up the idea of getting her teeth fixed first, before trust had been established and before she felt like she was healing, she probably wouldn't have come back. But once she felt more pulled together and atttractive, the logical next step was to fix her teeth, and so I brought it up at that point.

A young man who smoked PCP in college had, over the years, been treated for a misdiagnosed psychological disease with the extremely powerful drug Haldol. He still lived with his parents and his life was going nowhere. I usually give patients a hug at each session—this is a sort of trademark for me—but after a few goal-setting sessions, I admitted to this patient that he didn't smell so hot, and that hugging him wasn't very rewarding for me. He trusted me, and so didn't take offense; he wanted to please me, and so he started paying more attention to his personal hygiene.

Soon after that he began to look for employment, and one day he was looking for an excuse to get out of a planned interview. He wanted me to write him a note, and I refused. I told him to keep straightening his spine, take care of his own business. Because it came from me, he could hear this as constructive, not as an attack.

Invariably, the first goal I work with my patients on is *self-empowerment.* A lot of them don't think they need to be empowered, but the power they believe they have is really a straw house that will blow down in the next big wind. It is the kind of power that comes from anger and fear, and I want them to experience a power that is loving, kind, and compassionate.

I once treated the father of a well-known pro ballplayer. He was living indigent, relying on his successful son for handouts, although he himself had once been a star and had been his son's inspiration. We made goals that allowed him to feel that power and responsibility again, without fear. We made goals that enabled him to take back the mantle of leader of the tribe..

A male gang member, for example, sources his power from his relationships with his homeboys and his capacity to do violence and strike fear into the hearts of others. He needs this kind of power because he feels so powerless. So, we work to develop a new sense of power—one that comes from within, that is founded in peace and love instead of anger and violence. A young woman who has been sexually abused by a relative may feel most powerful when she is using her sexuality to attract men; we would work to move her away from that source of power and into a power that is more about who she is beneath it all.

After that initial 90-day period, we move on to other goals as determined in the treatment plan. Cognitive therapy teaches the patient to see how thinking patterns distort reality, and how that distortion of reality leads to symptoms such as anxiety and depression. The behavioral aspect of therapy breaks the connection between life situations and reactions to those situations. Behavioral therapy also involves training in methods for relaxing the mind and body, and helps the patient to use those methods during stressful situations.

Cognitive-behavioral therapy (CBT) was developed in the 1960s as a method for the treatment of depression. Since then, the majority of clinical research has shown us that this form of therapy is the most effective at treating the whole spectrum of psychological problems. Those who are treated with CBT are less likely to relapse than those treated with other methods, including drugs.

CBT is unique from other kinds of psychotherapy in several ways. Rather than the traditional paternalistic therapist-patient relationship, the interaction between healer and patient is reminiscent of coaching, teaching, tutoring, educating. Patients get homework assignments, including reading. (There is a need for culturally relevant readings for minorities.) It uses specific techniques to help patients stay in the present and move forward in a focused way, by working to alter attitudes, thoughts, ideas, beliefs, assumptions, mental images, self-talk, and ways of focusing their attention that hold them back. It involves an explicit treatment plan that is understood by both the therapist and the patient.

Therapy should go for no more than six to nine months, and it may be intermittent. You and your therapist will decide together when a break seems called for. During the course of those months, you will develop the skills and create the tools with which to work out your own problems. As you do this you will need the therapist less and less, and one day you'll realize: Hey, I can do this on my own now.

With my patients, once therapy is concluded and they have reached a healthier, more functional state, I tell them that they are free to call me if they need a nudge in the right direction. I also tell them *not* to call if they know, in their hearts, that this is something they can fix on their own. They almost never call. They are almost embarrassed to call, because they know that they can handle it themselves.

Chapter Ten

How Violent Media Both Help and Hurt

From the suffering of our people came rap.
—Louis Farrakhan

The celebration of violence, sex and consumer culture speaks more to the success of American free-market economics than it does to hip-hop's audience...Some of the most outrageously misogynist lyricists are also some of the most "conscious" when it comes to identifying and articulating the current crises in African-American culture.
—Bakeri Kitwana, author of *The Hip-Hop Generation: Young Blacks and the Crisis in African-American Culture*, as quoted at www.urbanthinktank.org

In 2003, I took part in the first National African-American Mental Health Summit in Washington, D.C. We gathered for several days to talk about the poor state of African-American mental health and what culturally relevant ways we could find to change it. During a lull in the action, one of the handful of white participants suggested that Dr. King Davis—the chair of the conference and a highly esteemed black man—do a "soft-shoe" to provide entertainment for the waiting attendees.

Most of us giggled, but the moment hit home for a lot of the black folks at that conference. We were all made aware that the stereotypes of African-Americans as performers and puppets for the white folks are still a part of the collective unconscious.

Black people performing for the pleasure of white people—it's been going on since slave days in America. Gatherings of slaves for dancing and singing were allowed on some plantations, but these gatherings were often for the entertainment of the "massas."

In slave days, white plantation owners would organize competitive dances for their slaves. Whichever slave could impress the white owners with their movement abilities the most would walk away with a prize, often a cake. Interestingly, the most popular competitive dance became known as the cakewalk—a parody on the part of the slaves of the white people's more "uppity" ways of moving and dancing. The slaves would hold the stiff upper-body comportment they saw in the white people's social dances, and they would simultaneously dance loose and wild leg movements from the dances of their African forefathers. The slaveowners came to enjoy watching these parodies of themselves. Everyone had fun, but still, at the end of the day, the slaves went home to their shacks, and got up the next day to toil for their masters' profit.

Today, black athletes and rap, soul, and R&B performers are hugely popular across the board. Hip-hop culture has been mainstreamed. Track suits, now the thing to wear for any occasion, were popularized by one of the first widely popular rap groups, RunDMC, back in the 1980s. A new stereotype has come from this mainstreaming of hip-hop culture: the non-black person adopting black speech, dress, and mannerisms. In Whoopi Goldberg's prime-time sitcom, "Whoopi," a young female character who is dating Whoopi's brother is a white girl who has strenuously taken on the stereotypical speech patterns and dress of a "sister."

The slang of hip-hop can be seen and heard coming from young people in all walks of life. Vast audiences gather to watch NBA teams comprised almost entirely of African-Americans, showcasing their native athletic ability for the pleasure of mostly white fans. In the late weeks of November 2003, rap artists occupied the top three slots on the Billboard charts.

In the world of popular music, African-Americans have carved a sizeable niche for themselves—through talent and hard work, but also by capitalizing on the popularity of violent gangsta rap.

It's sad to see how many African-American children think that their only way out of poverty is to make it big as a rap star or athlete.

Their chances of doing so are less than their chances of being hit by lightning—twice. And even if they do make it, they are at risk of being taken advantage of by powerful, savvy agents, managers, and recording companies. A lot of African-American success stories turn tragic because these young artists and athletes sign away their rights to people who don't necessarily have their best interest in mind.

Take Mariah Carey, for instance. She recently had a breakdown in the midst of a tour. She was decompensating, but the record company wanted her to push through it and finish her tour and stick with the terms of her contract. By and large, producers, record companies, and agents don't care about the psychological health of these talented artists.

Or poor Michael Jackson. This is a man who was obviously traumatized by celebrity at a very young age. He has not been able to heal. At best, he is a Peter Pan figure, a man-boy who never grew up and who chooses to surround himself with children, who has no concept of how to relate to people at an adult level, and who is becoming increasingly bizarre as he grows older. His bizarreness is all the more apparent because of the way in which he has altered his appearance. Unlike many celebrities who hide their trauma under glamorous clothing and the power that money buys, Michael wears his pain on the outside.

At worst, Michael Jackson may be a pedophile. Either way, he has managed to avoid causing trauma to others with his music. His music is brilliant when it is best, and at worst, it is harmless and danceable. The album that made him famous worldwide, "Thriller," was musically influential and respected, but since then his albums haven't sold well. Perhaps if he had tried harder to express his pain through his music, he might have been able to heal his wounds, and he would have matured as an artist.

There's R. Kelly, the R&B artist accused of having sexual relations with a minor girl and videotaping it. Dr. Dre was charged with assaulting seven police officers at the BRE Convention in New Orleans and was linked to the stabbing of a teenager there. Oprah Winfrey, Lil' Kim, and Mary J. Blige have spoken out about the traumas they suffered in their childhoods—as victims rather than as perpetrators—and of their efforts to heal themselves as adults.

Many years ago, I worked with African-American scholarship students at Penn State. They were given their grant money in a lump sum, and these girls thought they were rich, and they'd run out and get their nails done and had no money when the bills came due. The colleges get the African-American quota met so they can maintain state college status, but these kids need more guidance about how to handle money, because a lot of them have never had any. Many African-American musicians, rappers, athletes, and other entertainers are no different from these young girls.

Hip-Hop and Rap: Healers of Trauma or Retraumatization?

I have worked with black entertainers and athletes, many of whom have suffered considerable trauma since their early youth. I've seen a lot of them decompensating. I've seen these young people thrust into the limelight and given enormous amounts of money. They go wild, spending left and right, and they end up bankrupt. So much of their music focuses on the trappings of material wealth, the prestige lent by brand names.

Rap lyrics boast that they've made it out of the ghetto, but what comes through is ridiculous materialism. Rap lyrics by male artists boast of female conquest as a part of the rights and privileges they can now afford, now that they've made it big.

You know the Queen Bee known for (doin' it way big)
We take trips to Mekenos, Greece
just to shop, we don't stop (doin' it way big)
This is for my millionaire glub golfers
Comin up like Halle and Denzel, winnin' the Oscars
Y'all get y'all diamonds from Jacob, I ain't mad at ya
I get mine straight out the Kimberly Gold Mine in Africa
I smack niggaz 'cross the face with a Centurion Card
who don't believe I'm (doin' it way big)
In the Contintental T, magnolia B
.. (man, she doin' it way big)
I'm comin' through Hummer stuntin', and I'm frontin'
Workin' that LaBurke and Hermes bag
Only multi-millionaires who know about that

be like...(damn, she doin' it way big)
...Got all glass, Benz in all class
I do it big, my first kid gon' have a crib all brass
This is, exotic y'all, I got it y'all
Every color lizard watch from Scotty y'all
Private jets, Tiffany silverware sets
I got shit department stores ain't even get yet
I drop 30 or more in Christian Dior
They gotta close the store and let me shop some more
We go to Broadway plays in six white Rolls Royce
(now that's what you call doin' it way big)

...We greet our guests at the door
with champagne and cigars that read (doin' it way big)
Chrome on the doors, stone on the floors
Fourteen karat gold paint on the walls
We swim in pools with marble waterfalls
Ball baby or don't ball at all
My bathroom is Chanel, my bedroom Louis Vuitton
And office decorated in Ralph Lauren
I got a Versace couch and pillows I sleep on
With the matchin' robe and slippers, I beg to differ
LaPerla lingerie, 'cause it fits my body
Get with us, we know how to throw a party
And you can't get in, without a Queen Bee members only jacket
that reads (doin' it way big)

—Lil' Kim, "Doin' It Way Big"

Raising this kind of materialism to high status works against African-Americans. It fails to value the regular folks, the mothers and the fathers who struggle to do right by one another, their families, and their communities. This kind of music sends the message to children that they ought to strive for wealth and material possessions, rather than to be good wives, husbands, parents, friends, and members of the church and community. It presents a picture of impossible wealth that poor people can't identify with, but that is hard not to long for.

Are we supposed to feel proud of Lil' Kim for having such enormous wealth, because she is black? I don't. I don't want her representing me to the world.

I don't altogether blame artists like Lil' Kim, or the gangsta rappers who seek to make millions by penning violent, traumatizing lyrics and presenting themselves as killers to impressionable young people. Many of them come from great trauma themselves, and they are playing that trauma out in their music.

One of the most powerful ways humanity deals with trauma is through art. The alchemical process of transmuting hurt, sadness, or joy into a work of art that can communicate those emotions to others—and, hopefully, can provide a forum where those who view that art can identify and empathize with the artist's experience—is healing to both artist and viewer.

On the other hand, exposure to violence and extreme sexual content can be traumatizing or re-traumatizing. In some instances, this trauma is an integral part of the experience of the work of art. "Boyz In the Hood" and "Do The Right Thing" are both about the ways in which violence destroys African-American individuals, families, and communities, and their portrayal of that violence shook us deeply enough to leave us changed forever. Without that impact, art can't do what the best of it does best: change the world.

What the fuck's up!
DTP in this mother fucker
And for all y'all that don't like it
Do one thing, get the fuck back
'Cause all my niggaz is ready
Luda, 20, Fate, Shawna
Let's show these mutha fuckers how we disturb the peace
Get the fuck back, bitch
[shooting and screaming in the background]

Fuck that!
Get the fuck back!
Luda make your skull crack
Tuck that
Bitch, your whole town's on my nutsack

Cuff that
Put it in your weed, nigga, puff that
What's that
People gon' die tonight

—Ludacris, "Get The Fuck Back" (featuring Fate Wilson, I-20, Shawna)

Either the man who wrote these lyrics is in pain, or he is shamelessly exploiting the public's taste for violent entertainment. Whatever the reasons for it, these lyrics are traumatizing. They don't help. They incite violence.

We don't have to do things this way; we can be more positive and still accurately describe our experience. LL Cool J, one of the most popular and long-lived rap stars around, keeps it positive. He suffered trauma in his childhood, too. He was from the projects, too. But he has managed to heal himself.

Some African-American rap artists are stepping up to the plate and acknowledging their pain, and they are attempting to clean up their work. The rest are in denial. As a result, they are creating trauma in young people, revictimizing them, and creating the wrong kind of role models for a culture that desperately needs the right ones.

Before the LA Riots, before gangsta rap became popular in the mid-1990s, rap and hip-hop were more positive. Hip-hop parties were positive events where young people could come together and feel unity and celebrate. The hip-hop movement was strongest in New York City and along the East Coast, and so-called East Coast rap was, by and large, about healing, political activism, and unity amongst African-Americans. The music and words encouraged youth to remember their roots and better themselves and their communities:

You spend a buck in the 80's, what you get is a preacher
Forgivin' this torture of the system that brought 'cha
I'm on a mission and you got that right
Addin' fuel to the fire, punch to the fight
Many have forgotten what we came here for
Never knew or had a clue, so you're on the floor
Just growin not knowin about your past
now you're lookin' pretty stupid while you're shakin' your ass

Mind over matter, mouth in motion
Can't deny cause I'll never be quiet
Let's start this right

Some people fear me when I walk this way
Some come near me, some run away
Some people take heed to every word I say
Some wanna build a posse, some stay away
Some people think that we plan to fail
Wonder why we go under or go to yail
Some ask us why we act the way we act
Without lookin' how long they kept us back

...Yes you if I bore you, I won't ignore you
I'm sayin things that they say I'm not supposed to
Give you pride that you may not find
If you're blind about your past then ill point behind
Kings, Queens, warriors, lovers
People proud, sisters and brothers
It's the biggest fear, suckers get tears
When we can top their best idea

...Our solution, mind revolution
Mind over matter, mouth in motion
Corners don't sell it, no you can't buy it
Can't defy it cause I'll never be quiet
Let's start this right

Our solution, mind revolution
Can't sell it, no you can't buy it in a potion
You lie about the life that you wanted to try
Tellin' me about a head, you decided to fly
Another brother with the same woes that you face
But you shot with the same hands, you fall from grace
Every brother should be every brother's keeper
But you shot with your left while your right was on your beeper

...As the world turns, it's a terrible waste
To see the stupid look stuck on your face
Timebomb alarm for the world, just try it
Known to all zones as the one man riot
I'm on a mission to set you straight
Children, it's not too late
Explain to the world when it's plain to see
To be what the world doesn't want us to be...

—Public Enemy, "Rightstarter (Message to a Black Man)"

Violence and Sex in Rap Lyrics: Gratuitous or Necessary?

Great rap music brings listeners more deeply into the experience of African-American youth and of their hopes and dreams than any documentary, scholarly work, or newspaper article. There is no arguing that even the most violent rap lyrics can be remarkably poetic, but those lyrics can be so harsh and hateful that they bring out more anger than they heal.

I get tapes doin' times, stop niggaz like grapes makin wine
Five CDs with mad rhymes
Don't hit me with that positive shit, I know you lyin'
You really wanna stop niggaz from dyin'? Stop niggaz from tryin'
'Cuz I ain't really got that time to waste
and I thought I told you to get these fuckin' bums out my face
Lookin atchu in your grill, I might be nice to cut
Once I split ya ass in two, you'll be twice as butt
Yeah, you right, I know ya style—PUSSY 'cuz I'm fuckin' it
Since we all right here, you hold my dick while he suckin' it
MOTHERFUCKER, don't you know you'll never come near me
Shove ya head up ya ass, have you seein' shit clearly
Never heard that D be runnin', 'cuz D be gunnin'
I beat my dick and bust off in ya eye so you can see me comin'
Empty clips and shells are what I leave behind
and if they get me with the joint, they hit me with a three-to-nine

—DMX, "Where the Hood At"

The question remains: how do we hang on to the transformative, the cathartic, the smack-upside-the-head epiphanies that great art has to offer, without making the problem of trauma worse in the process?

Those who would censor the media and the arts talk a lot about *gratuitous violence* and *gratuitous sex.* The dictionary on my desk defines *gratuitous* as simply 1. given free of charge 2. uncalled-for. This word doesn't do much to help us discriminate between the art that heals and the art that hurts.

Some would argue that lyrics that are written for the purpose of raising consciousness will inevitably become fuel for fires of hatred. People find what they are looking for. When a person who is peace-minded listens to a violent rap, he thinks, "This is a statement against violence, a warning." When a person who is violent-minded listens to the same rap, he might hear it as a call to violent action.

Dear diary: today I hit a nigga with a torch
Shot him on his face and watched him die on his front porch
Left his family heartbroken
Flashbacks of him laying there bleeding with his eyes open
I can't put the shit behind me
I'm know I'm here somewhere, but I can't find me
I used to be a drug dealer
On the fo'reala
Now I'm a born killer
And it ain't no changing me
It used to be hard, but now it ain't no thing to me
To go up to a nigga's house
Put a pistol in his mouth and blow his fucking brains out

—Scarface, "Diary of a Madman"

We can't make this distinction unless we acknowledge the historical roots of rap. When violence or sex is reflected in the lyrics, are those violent or sexual words only there to shock, or do they have historical validity? Are they meant to elevate consciousness, or incite riots? "Don't deny the roots and state the craft is criminal," writes black journalist Bakari Akil II.

The Roots of Modern African-American Arts

Traditional African dance and music served many purposes. They were an integral part of culture, just as they are in modern African-American life. There were social dances that brought men and women together. There were recreational dances, and there were sacred dances.

Sacred dances were often about possession—about a god taking over the body of the dancer and speaking through it. Chanting, drumming, and dancing combined would bring the participants into an altered state of consciousness, removing them from reality.

Today's African-American youth needs this escape hatch; it's far healthier than drugs, violence, and sex. Unfortunately, much of the music young blacks listen to and dance to celebrate these very things.

Slaves learned Christian hymns on plantations. They learned songs like "Amazing Grace," the sound of which "saved a wretch like me." The music that the Africans brought with them had a much more positive message. They did not reflect degradation; they reflected pride, and the slaves managed to hold on to that pride in the music they continued to create.

Slaves also used music and other native arts to communicate that which they did not want the whites to know. In slave days, grandmothers would sew beautiful quilts,which that were actually maps of the Underground Railroad, to hang outside their windows. Drumming was used to relay messages. In fact, drumming was outlawed among slaves after the Cato Conspiracy, a slave revolt that was organized in 1739 through the use of drum signals.

Blackface and Minstrel Shows

Everyone has heard the stereotypes: white men can't dance, white men can't jump. Of course there are exceptions to these rules. I've seen white men do some spectacular dancing, and I've also seen black men who can't dance a step. But it does seem that something in the African-American genetic makeup enhances their ability to move rhythmically to music, and to move quickly and jump high.

If you were to take a randomly selected crowd of black people and a randomly selected crowd of people of other races, you could bet on more of the black people being able to either sing, dance, or jump well enough to be considered entertaining. This isn't racism, it's just the truth, and it has been both a blessing and a curse.

African-American entertainment first became the rage during the era of minstrel shows, between 1845 and 1900. Up to 50 black performers would travel with a show that depicted African-Americans in one of two stereotypical ways: as a vain dandy in stylish clothing, or as—in the words of dance historian Bob Boross—a "slow, shuffling idiot." There was banter, burlesque, singing, and dancing, and no doubt these shows were among the most entertaining stuff there was to be seen at the time.

Before that time, white performers imitated black dance moves, blackening their faces with burnt cork. In 1828, white dancer Thomas Rice came up with a dance called the Jump Jim Crow—a dance based on the movement of a crippled slave. The Jump Jim Crow was enormously popular all over the world.

We haven't come that far from the days of minstrel shows—of all of the hugely gifted black artists and entertainers and athletes who America watched with awe and respect, but who were still not allowed to go to the same hotels or restaurants or to drink from the same water fountains as whites.

One of the most fascinating movies ever made on this topic was Spike Lee's film *Bamboozled.* According to Salon.com's Andrew O'Hehir, "Lee's title is drawn from a speech by Malcolm X that he sneaks into one of his montage scenes (as seen in his own 1992 film). 'You've been hoodwinked,' Malcolm tells his Harlem audience. 'You've been had. You've been took. You've been led astray, run amuck. You've been bamboozled.' Is this a different way of expressing Junebug's [the African-American nightclub performer father of the movie's main character, Delacroix] cynical maxim: 'Every nigger is an entertainer'? Is there no difference between the obsequious clowning of Stephin Fetchit and a millionaire gangsta rapper?"

The film is about Delacroix, a black TV studio executive who is exhorted by his white boss, Dunwitty, to come up with a groundbreaking, sensational new program. Delacroix creates a "New Millennium Minstrel Show," featuring the same stereotypes that were featured in original minstrelsy—including a dandy (Mantan) and a buffoon (Sleep N' Eat). The show is a runaway hit, but a gang of black activists—the Mau-Maus, led by the brother of Delacroix's assistant, Sloan—is so angered by it that they take drastic action that ends up crumbling the whole operation.

Earlier in his review, O'Hehir tells us that *Bamboozled's* imagery of *shuffling servants, kerchief-clad mammies, grinning cartoon "pickaninnies" and jive-ass pimps is almost overwhelmingly painful to watch. Lee's point, as I read it, is that all Americans, white, black and otherwise, have been indoctrinated by relentless decades of these stereotypes. The classic blackface minstrel shows of the 19th century, and most subsequent ideas about blacks, were driven by envy almost as much as contempt. Black caricatures like Mantan and Sleep 'N Eat are ignorant, lazy and unlucky (as Delacroix explains to the delighted Dunwitty), but they're also free of the restraints and obligations of white society. These depictions of blackness, shaped by a poisoned history that is neither long in the past nor far below the surface, have seduced blacks and whites in different but interrelated ways. We ignore that history at our peril.*

Lee doesn't cut the Mau Maus much slack, either. O'Hehir writes:

Lee paints them as only slightly less ridiculous caricatures of blackness, in their gold chains, 'do rags and baggy FUBU jeans, than Mantan and Sleep 'N Eat. Sloan's brother Julius (rapper Mos Def), who now calls himself Big Black Africa, is the group's leader, and the best he can do by way of philosophy is to insist, "We talking about getting free in America, USA, KKK, all that shit." Like everybody else, Big Black's real agenda is to get on TV; if the Monkees and the Partridge Family could get their own shows, he asks Sloan, why can't the Mau Maus? The band's major militant insight, fueled by plenty of ganja and bottles of Da Bomb [a brand of beer sold in a bomb-shaped bottle], *is that the letter "c" must be removed from the word "black."*

In the early 1990s, West Coast rappers wanted a piece of the action. They capitalized on the publicity created by the riots, and gangsta rap was born. East Coast rappers saw how rich the gangsta rappers became, and they followed suit with similarly traumatizing lyrics. Feuds between East and West Coast rappers became a common topic in gangsta rap music. Those rap stars who refused to heal got involved in feuds that sometimes culminated in murder. Tupac Shakur and Notorious B.I.G. were two of the best-known casualties of this pointless feuding.

In slave days, and before that in Africa, dance and music were safe places for men to compete, one-upping each other with their acrobatic abilities. Dance was a safe mating ritual, allowing women to show their seductive sides in a protected setting. The art of "signifying," where people who were downtrodden used language to trick those who were doing the treading, has long been another healthy form of competition between African-Americans: who could outdo the others with the most devastating insult to the white folks, without the white folks catching on?

Another variation on this is known variously as "playing the dozens," "capping," "cracking," "dissing," "ranking," "ribbing," and "serving," where two people hurl insults and wisecracks at one another, usually in front of an appreciative audience. Playing the dozens is the source of the now-tired "Your momma is so fat…" lead-in.

Today, these displays of verbal agility, these battles of the wits, have given way to real threats, to battles with bullets where people die for saying the wrong thing. In this environment, we have confused the line between the kind of healthy competition that makes men men, and the kind of deadly rivalries that show more cowardice and small-mindedness than real power.

Hip-hop is an American cultural movement that has its roots in African music and movement. It is much more than music, although music is one of its most important aspects. Graffiti and breakdancing—an important element of what is today known as hip-hop dance—are also elements of hip-hop.

In the late 1960s and 1970s, a young DJ named Clive Campbell—Kool Herc to most who knew him—developed a way to extend the instrumental 'breaks' on the records he spun. He would use two copies of the same album, on adjacent turntables, and would artfully spin both records to lengthen these sections of the music. Dancers would come out to show their best moves during these breaks—hence, the term "breakdancing." These dancers, who came to be known as "B-boys," created their daring moves from a combination of traditional African dance and a Brazilian martial art called *capoeira.*

The steps were created, performed, and passed along in the streets. The influence of martial arts was partly due to the influence of breakdancing pioneers who were members of New York and Los Angeles street gangs. Locking, popping, and uprock were all elements of early hip-hop dance, created by these first B-Boys. At block parties, house parties, and clubs, DJs began to speak rhythmically over the breaks in the music they played, an imitation of Caribbean music that gave birth to what we now know as rap.

At the same time, graffiti became a popular form of self-expression in the newly developing hip-hop culture. A mail courier named Vic would leave his "tag"—Vic 156, his name and courier number—on all the subways and buses he rode on his route. Others soon followed suit, and graffiti became an art form that was widely reviled as vandalism.

Graffiti was a perfect form of expression for disenfranchised young people: it was anonymous, illegal, but very, very public, and made their presence known in their "territory." In the very act of expressing themselves, graffiti artists thumb their noses at the powers that be. The various styles of graffiti lettering—or "piecing"—such as bubble, computer style, and wild style, were passed along much as dance steps were passed along. Like hip-hop dance and music, graffiti continues to hold its appeal in the less socioeconomically privileged segments of African-American culture.

In 1986, RunDMC released a hip-hop version of Aerosmith's song "Walk This Way." It quickly climbed the charts, and there began the huge popularity of hip-hop music. Since then, rap and hip-hop have been a constant presence on the pop charts, MTV, and the mass media.

Funk and R&B—also made primarily by African-American performers—are a part of the foundation of today's music industry, as well. In fact, just about every kind of American popular music, including rock and roll, jazz, and blues, originated in African-American culture.

Freestyle rappers still compete in clubs and on the streets. There is a lot of posturing and signifying in rap today, even in the more "positive" hip-hop music. The language of gangsta rap is still there, but it's referring to battles of words and wits instead of guns and knives.

I'm kinda like a soldier, see I told ya
When I pick up the mic I'm-a hold ya
captive, a mack-tive, I'll make sure I'll track it
L'll speak a cell a sneak as your backs' gettin' weaker
I freak the beat and get sheiker
Rule over King, you're too over-eager
You're tryin' to make a move for
I'm-a prove you're ridiculious
I think he was jealous and in the mood for an ass-kickin'
When you mess with, the man with the plan
mic in his hand and a fresh skit
R-O-U-G-H-E-R, ROUGHER!! So here we are
Face to face, mic to mic, man to man
While your battle ship is sinkin' in quicksand
Strappin' to the bottom like a two-ton anchor
And break, pull the rope, point blank, I'm a sniper
Rapper like a pack, step on 'em like a mack
My DJ Cut-Creator scratch a record like a cat
E at my side with pride who got a bigger rep
Shh... smoke the mic like a cigarette
Every puff is rough I pull, kill a bull
One toke, your crews' a joke
I run through rappers like runnin' through rubber holes is
Nigga, I'm comin' up roses
Step back—I got the title—bear-witness to a dope recital
I've killed many men my friend and I'm-a do it again and
again and again
Cause it gets no rougher

YouknowI'msayin'? I'm rulin' this game
It don't get no rougher...peace—LL Cool J

—LL Cool J, "It Gets No Rougher"

Feuds between rappers are often addressed in their music—still playing the dozens, but with a deadly edge.

Ain't got no motherfuckin' friends
That's why I fucked yo' bitch
You fat motherfucker
(Take money)
West side
Bad Boy killaz

...Fuck your bitch and the clique you claim
West side when we ride
Come equipped with game
You claim to be a player
But I fucked your wife
We bust on Bad Boyz' niggaz
Fucked for life
Plus, Puffy tryin' to see me
Weak hearts I rip
Biggie Smallz and Junior M.A.F.I.A.
Some mark ass bitches
We keep on comin
While we runnin for ya jewels

... Go ask your homie how I leave ya
Cut your young ass up
Leave you in pieces
Now be deceased
Lil' Kim
Don't fuck around with real Gs
Quick to snatch your ugly ass off the street
So fuck peace
I let them niggas know it's on for life
So let the West side ride tonight hahaa
Bad Boy murdered on wax and killed
Fuck with me and get ya caps peeled

...Grab your glocks when you see Tupac
Call the cops when you see Tupac (uh)
Who shot me, but ya punks didn't finish
Now ya bout to feel the wrath of a menace
Nigga, I hit 'em up!

—Tupac Shakur, "hit 'em up"

Work It: Women In Hip-Hop Culture

The devaluation of women is another serious issue in hip-hop culture. Women are portrayed in hip-hop and rap videos and on album covers as nothing more than sexual objects, among the many objects that are easily claimed by newly rich rap stars. Rap lyrics portray women as prizes won through the conquest of another man—spoils of war, to whom anything can be done. Their desire to participate isn't usually part of the scene. Female rap artists like Lil' Kim and Missy "Misdemeanor" Elliott attempt to equalize the playing field with their own sexually explicit lyrics, which portray them as the same kind of sexual adventurers as their male counterparts:

I'd like to get to know ya so I could show ya
Put the pussy on ya like I told ya
Gimme all your numbers so I could phone ya
Your girl actin' stank then call me over
Not on the bed, lay me on your sofa
Phone before you come, I need to shave my cha-cha
You do or you don't or you will or won't ya
Go downtown and eat it like a vulture
See my hips and my tips, don't ya
See my ass and my lips, don't ya
Lost a few pounds and my whips for ya
This the kinda beat that go ra-ta-ta
Ra-ta-ta-ta-ta-ta-ta-ta-ta-ta
Sex me so good I say blah-blah-blah
Work it, I need a glass of water
Boy, oh, boy, it's good to know ya

...If you a fly gal get your nails done
Get a pedicure, get your hair did
Boy, lift it up, let's make a toast-a
Let's get drunk, that's gon' bring us closer
Don't I look like a Halle Berry poster
See the Belvedere playin' tricks on ya
Girlfriend wanna be like me, never
You won't find a bitch that's even better
I make you hot as Las Vegas weather
Listen up close while I take it backwards
I'm not a prostitute, but I could give you what you want

—Missy Elliott, "Work It"

Missy Elliott's music is hardly traumatizing, especially to young adults who are already knowledgeable about sex. But it does celebrate sex without the kind of love that creates a foundation for family and community life.

Moving Away From *Destructive Stereotypes*

In an article posted at www.alternet.com, Earl Ofari Hutchinson writes:

In the past few years, a rogue's list of rappers have been assaulted, murdered or run afoul of the law. They revel in the bad actor lifestyle and play hard on the us-versus-them volcanic rage of many young blacks. They reap a king's ransom from exploiting the violent, outlaw image of black life. Many young black men reinforce the damaging racial stereotypes by aping and exalting the thuggish bluster and behavior of gangster rappers...I challenge blacks to stop aiding and abetting their own shove to the netherworld of the American economy by reinforcing the destructive stereotypes about themselves.

—Earl Ofari Hutchinson, "Are Young Black Males America's Job Untouchables?" AlterNet, www.alternet.com, November 17, 2003.

If African-Americans want to heal, they need to stop providing both marketplace and material for media that traumatize and re-traumatize children and adults. We need to send a message to gangsta rappers and others who would promote violence and hatred that they are hurting their own. They may be laughing all the way to the bank, but they are walking on the future of African-American children as they go.

Chapter Eleven

The Gifts of Trauma

As I wrote in the Introduction a couple of hundred pages ago, you are formally invited to become a part of the healing journey. Not only are you invited, you are needed. As we've all heard it said, if you aren't a part of the solution, you're part of the problem, and high time has come for solutions to the problems of traumatized people. Unresolved trauma is a highly concentrated poison that doesn't restrict itself to the soul and mind of one person. We all must share in the burden of releasing that pain.

Use what you have learned from these pages to advocate for yourself (if you are a victim of trauma), to forgive yourself for your own mistakes, and to heal.

If you are a therapist, I hope that you feel better equipped to offer culturally relevant solutions to your African-American patients and other minorities.

If you are a policymaker or clergyperson, I hope you will be able to better support your community from here on forward.

If you are a mother or a father, remember that it's up to you to prepare your children to be as resilient as possible, and that it's okay to ask for help in doing so. Draw on your clan, and if you don't have one, create one.

If you are a human being, remember that you come into contact with traumatized people virtually every day. By simply listening and being open to their pain, you help lift a burden that weighs us all down.

Taking Back Our Pride, Taking Back Our Communities

The Million Man March was organized by Minister Louis Farrakhan, the leader of the Nation of Islam. Minister Farrakhan is a controversial figure—his statements about Jews and whites have caused him to be labeled a racist—but the intention of the march proved larger than his reputation. Hundreds of thousands of black men swarmed onto the Washington Mall to hear speeches and music and to pledge themselves, in Minister Farrakhan's words, as "sober, disciplined, committed, dedicated, inspired Black men" meeting for "a day of atonement."

Then-President William Jefferson Clinton spoke to the crowd. He pointed out that as a nation, we have allowed ourselves to become complacent about racial inequality, despite the facts: that African-Americans earn, on average, 60 percent of what whites earn; half of African-American children grow up in poverty; nearly one in three black men in their 20s is either in prison or on probation. From President Clinton's speech:

...Today's march is also about pride and dignity and respect. But after a generation of deepening social problems that disproportionately impact black Americans, it is also about black men taking renewed responsibility for themselves, their families and their communities.

It's about saying "no" to crime and drugs and violence. It's about standing up for atonement and reconciliation. It's about insisting that others do the same and offering to help them. It's about the frank admission that, unless black men shoulder their load, no one else can help them or their brothers, their sisters and their children escape the hard, bleak lives that too many of them still face.

...No good house was ever built on a bad foundation. Nothing good ever came of hate. So let us pray today that all who march and all who speak will stand for atonement, for reconciliation, for responsibility.

Let us pray that those who have spoken for hatred and division in the past will turn away from that past and give voice to the true message of those ordinary Americans who march.

...Today, we face a choice. One way leads to further separation and bitterness and more lost futures. The other way—the path of

courage and wisdom—leads to unity, to reconciliation, to a rich opportunity for all Americans to make the most of the lives God gave them.

This moment, in which the racial divide is so clearly out in the open, need not be a setback for us. It presents us with a great opportunity and we dare not let it pass us by.

In the past, when we've had the courage to face the truth about our failure to live up to our own best ideals, we've grown stronger, moved forward, and restored proud American optimism. At such turning points, America moved to preserve the Union and abolish slavery, to embrace women's suffrage, to guarantee basic legal rights to America without regard to race under the leadership of President Johnson.

...White America must understand and acknowledge the roots of black pain. It began with unequal treatment, first in law, and later in fact. African Americans, indeed, have lived too long with a justice system that in too many cases has been, and continues to be, less than just.

...On the other hand, blacks must understand and acknowledge the roots of white fear in America.

There is a legitimate fear of the violence that is too prevalent in our urban areas and often, by experience or at least what people see on the news at night, violence for those white people too often has a black face.

It isn't racist for a parent to pull his or her child close when walking through a high crime neighborhood. Or, to wish to stay away from neighborhoods where innocent children can be shot in school or standing at bus stops by thugs driving by with assault weapons or toting handguns...It isn't racist for parents to recoil in disgust when they read about a national survey of gang members saying that two thirds of them feel justified in shooting someone simply for showing them disrespect.

For most black Americans still do work hard, care for their families, pay their taxes and obey the law. Often, under circumstances which are far more difficult than those their white counterparts face.

Imagine how you would feel if you were a young parent in your twenties with a young child living in a housing project, working somewhere for $5 an hour with no health insurance, passing, every day, people on the street selling drugs, making one hundred times what you make. Those people are the real heroes of America today and we should recognize that.

So, we all have a stake in solving these common problems together. It is, therefore, wrong for white Americans to do what they have done too often, simply to move further away from the problems and support policies that will only make them worse.

It has been nearly a decade, and the fervor of that consciousness-raising gathering has long since died down. Not much has changed since that march. Black people are still suffering disproportionately. Black men are still rejecting responsibility. Black women are still stuck in dead-end situations, raising children on their own. Black children are still subjected to traumatizing circumstances day in and day out, and will—unless something is done on their behalf—most likely perpetuate the cycle of trauma.

President Clinton touched upon the notion that black pain needs to be acknowledged, but he also stated that while African-Americans have been victimized, we need to move beyond victim status and take responsibility for ourselves, our families, and our communities. As we move towards an acceptance of the pervasive effects of trauma that are unique to our people because of our history, the acceptance of our own responsibility for healing that trauma will be a natural outgrowth of that shift.

I do not mean to imply that healing black trauma is completely up to black people. Healing happens best when we all see one another as human, rather than as sharply divided along lines of race, gender, or belief. The most basic tools for that healing—compassion, empathy, love, and an open heart—are within the scope of every human being, regardless of their skin color.

It is important, however, to *offer our help to others who are in distress in ways that are culturally relevant.* This is where the race card comes in. With this book, I have attempted to outline such culturally relevant ways to aid African-Americans who are perpetuating the cycle of trauma in their families and their communities.

Pain Should Be Shared

A young friend of my daughter's recently had her first baby. During her pregnancy, she went to a prenatal exercise class. She became acquainted with most of the women who regularly attended the class.

Then, tragedy struck. The baby of one of the women in the class—let's call her Delia—was stillborn. There was no warning, no problem, no indication of anything wrong until a routine ultrasound showed that the baby's heart had stopped beating.

My daughter's friend had not been close to Delia. They were acquaintances only. Although she was deeply saddened by what had happened, she did not call or reach out to Delia in any other way after the baby's death. "I told myself that she needed time," she told me, "and then, it seemed awkward to call. What if she was ready to stop talking about it? What if by calling I re-opened or poured salt on her wounds?" And so she never called.

A few months later, my daughter's friend was grocery shopping with her baby. Her little son was sitting happily in her cart, babbling and drooling. She saw Delia slowly pushing her cart through the aisles, her eyes big as saucers, obviously still mourning her loss. She looked awful. She had gained weight, and looked as though she had just rolled out of bed after a poor night's sleep.

"I panicked," my daughter's friend told me. "I suddenly was convinced that seeing my baby would hurt her too much. I didn't know what I would say. I bent my head and made a point of not meeting her eyes. I know she saw me. She must have felt like a leper. Now I know that I wasn't scared for her, I was scared for myself. I couldn't stand to think of what her experience had been like. I was afraid to go there.

"I wish I had had the courage to meet her gaze and let her see my baby if she wanted. I wish I had been okay with the possibility that she might completely break down crying right there in the store, for everyone to see, and that I could sit with her all the way through it, maybe right there on the floor with people pushing their carts past us. I wish that those people would have been okay with it, too, not gawking but opening to the presence of pain in such a workaday place. Not even asking, 'What's wrong?' or 'What happened?' but just allowing the pain."

Every day, survivors of trauma are made to feel like outcasts. When they need support the most, they are ostracized, as though their pain were contagious.

Well, it *is* contagious, and that is all right. Pain should be shared. The sharing of pain lessens the burden on everyone. It maintains our awareness of the problems in the world—the problems that require our attention and work to be healed. When we refuse to share in the pain of others, we are preserving our own little comfortable sphere of existence for the time being, but this happens to the detriment of the clan and of the world.

How often are those who are in pain told to "get over it," given platitudes such as "everything will be fine," or "tomorrow's another day," or "it was meant to be"? Too often. Platitudes are our way of avoiding the issue, of doing enough time as the comforter to feel okay about ourselves without really giving over any part of ourselves. Then we race off to our own lives, relieved that we can check that off our lists for today. We avoid, we bury our heads, and the problems that cause so much pain to the few continue to be ignored by the many. Trauma is too often sugar-coated or Hollywood-ized in Western culture. "It was just like a movie!" is one of the most common things I hear from people describing what it was like to be in a traumatic situation. But there is no happy Hollywood ending, no credits rolling, no filing out of the theater at the end when we are dealing with real trauma.

The most important thing to do when we encounter someone who has been traumatized is to simply sit with that person in an open and loving way. We can do this for anyone, be it a stranger, friend, or relative. Sounds simple, but it has become all but impossible for most modern people. No one has told us how to do this, or even that we should.

There might be conversation, there might not. Remember to breathe deeply and relax. There is no formula. The key is to be absolutely present and attentive to the person in pain.

Pain is contagious. We have to allow this. Refusing to let the pain of others into our own bodies, minds, and souls sickens us almost as much as being the one who has been traumatized. Pain has its gifts; anyone who has given birth to a child knows this first-hand. Most trauma survivors who get the help they need to move towards healing admit that they have learned or gained something from their experience—both the trauma itself and the healing process. They say that the pain they have gone through has, in the end, enriched their lives immeasurably.

The more of someone's pain we are willing to absorb, the faster both of us will heal. We just have to be willing to go there, to really feel it. There is no shortcut, no avoiding this. Pain is a part of the human experience.

Pain that goes unacknowledged will grow and fester until we can no longer avoid it. Acknowledged, that pain is transformed into a healing energy.

In our culture, people in pain are looked upon as either victims or malingerers. Victims are seen as helpless pawns, decimated by powers greater than themselves; malingerers hang onto their pain and try to share it with every last soul they can get near. A truly healing approach to trauma sees trauma survivors neither as victims or malingerers, but as people who are in pain, *right now,* who need support, *right now.*

Victims are empowered by this approach. Malingerers only bombard others with their pain because they feel that no one is really listening. Once listened to and fully acknowledged, they can stop.

Think of your childhood. Did you ever tell a parent that something was hurting you or scaring you, only to be told to get over it or that it didn't really matter? You most likely went on being scared or hurt, and on top of that you didn't feel heard. The need to be heard—really and truly heard, not just given a chance to say something—is universal. Try this: next time someone tells you that something is hurtful or scary to them, simply acknowledge what they have said. If your child comes in and tells you she's scared of the dark, don't tell her that there's nothing to be scared of. Tell her, "Yes, the dark can be scary. I know it's hard to be scared." Don't fix it, or try to squash it. See what happens. You'll most likely see her breathe a big sigh of relief. *Mommy understands. Daddy understands.* That's half the battle.

Those who suffer the pain of trauma have a hard task at hand, too. They must be willing to feel their own pain and share it with others. Although whatever traumatized them is not their fault, it is their *responsibility* to get whatever help they need to heal. They must take time to allow their pain to come forth, to hold it, to acknowledge it. They must be willing to accept the help and support of others, and to reject seemingly easy fixes: addiction, denial, blaming. All of these responses to trauma end up perpetuating it.

This is not a brief process or an easy one. But it is the foundation for the healing of trauma at both the individual and community levels.

What To Do Next

We need to do what it takes to heal and to claim our power, because this will provide a safety net for future generations, and a springboard for healing in our communities.

If you are a trauma survivor, seek out help. Do it today. You can start by contacting A Gift From Within, an international organization for trauma survivors; they can be found at www.giftfromwithin.org/. Look in your local phone book and call some therapists in your area. Refer back to Chapter Nine for guidelines on how to choose a therapists—look for someone who does cognitive/behavioral therapy, and if you can, find a therapist who has dealt a lot with trauma.

If you are a therapist, chances are good that most of your clients have been touched by trauma.Try to attune yourself to the presence of post-traumatic stress in your patients. If you haven't studied cogitive/behavioral approaches, do some reading or continuing education courses on this topic. Attend trainings, seminars, and presentations on culturally sensitive and culturally relevant therapy. Talk to your colleagues about what you have learned.

If you are a policymaker or clergyperson, encourage the formation of clans and lasting interrelationships between individuals and groups. Help your flock to embrace a healthy way of life. Use your influence to help families better parent their children, to break the cycle of trauma.

If you are a mother or a father—especially if you were traumatized by your own parents—do whatever it takes to avoid passing that trauma on to your own children. Prepare them to face trauma in their own lives. Look into parenting classes if you need extra support. New mothers may want to contact attachment parenting groups, such as Attachment Parenting International at:

www.attachmentparenting.org/, or Parenting Web at www.parentingweb.com/ap/ap_index.htm. If you have any midwives or birth support networks in your area, they may know of parenting education and support groups that promote attachment parenting.

As a clinician, one of my favorite mantras has always been: *empowerment through education and awareness.* When we take the time to become educated and when we stop, take a breath, and become aware of what is going on both outside of us and within us, we become powerful. I hope that this book has served the purpose of raising your awareness and improving your education regarding the role of trauma in creating some of mankind's most pressing problems.

When we become powerful, we are not necessarily going to be protected against trauma. Virtually everyone I know has had the experience of knowing two kinds of people: the one who constantly worries about every possible bad thing that could happen, and the one who strides forth into each day without worry or fear. Neither of these individuals is any more or less likely to be a trauma victim. Bad things happen to all kinds of people. The powerful ones, the fearless ones, are the ones who are capable of confronting those traumas. They stand firm in who they are and what they believe in when trauma strikes.

They feel their pain just like anyone else, but then, they *heal.*

Endnotes

Blau JR, Blau PM, "The cost of inequality: Metropolitan structure and violent crime," Am Soc Rev 47;114-117.

Boross, Bob, "African-American Contributions to Theatrical Dance," compiled from "Image of Perfection: the Freestyle Dance of Matt Maddox,"
www.theatredance.com

Carlie, Mike, Ph.D., "Into the Abyss: A Personal Journey Into The World of Street Gangs," available at
http://courses.smsu.edu/mkc096f/gangbook/Preface/author.htm#©

Cecil H, Matson SC, "Psychological functioning and family discord among African-American adolescent females with and without a history of childhood sexual abuse,"
Child Abuse Negl 2001 Jul;25(7):973-88.

Dimitriou T, Maser-Gluth C, Remer T, "Adrenocortical activity in healthy children is associated with fat mass,"
Am J Clin Nutr 2003 Mar;77(3):731-6.

Everly GS, Mitchell JT, "Critical incident stress management: a new era and standard of care in crisis intervention," 2nd ed., Ellicott City, MD:Chevron Publishing Corporation.

Ferrari AM, "The impact of culture upon child rearing practices and definitions of maltreatment,"
Child Abuse Negl 2002 Aug 26;8:793-813.

Floyd, Samuel A., Jr., The Power of Black Music: Interpreting its History from Africa to the United States,

Oxford University Press, London:1995.

Fullerton CS, Ursano RI, eds.; Post-traumatic Stress Disorder: The Victim's Guide to Healing and Recovery,
New York: The Crossroad Publishing Company.

Herman, Judith L, Trauma and Recovery, Basic Books,
New York NY: 1992.

Hoschl C, Hajek T, "Hippocampal damage mediated by corticosteroids—a neuropsychiatric research challenge,"
Eur Arch Psychiatry Clin Neurosci 2001;251 Suppl 2:I181-8.

Lee AL, Ogle WO, Sapolsky RM, "Stress and depression: possible links to neuron death in the hippocampus,"
Bipolar Disord 2002 Apr;4(2):117-28.

Lutenbacher M, "Relationships between psychosocial factors and abusive parenting attitudes in low-income single mothers,"
Nurse Res 2002 May-June;51(3):158-67.

Murchison, Carl, History of Psychology in Autobiography, Vol. 1, p. 123-33; Clark University Press, Worcester MA:1930.

No authors listed, African-American Voices of Triumph:
Perseverance, Time-Life Books, Alexandria VA: 1993.

No authors listed, "Race/ethnicity, gender, socioeconomic status—research exploring their effects on child health: a subject review,"
Pediatrics, Vol 105, Number 6, June 2000, p. 1349-1351.

Ochberg, Frank M, International Handbook of Traumatic Stress Syndromes,
Plenum Press, New York NY:1993.

Penza KM, Heim C, Nemeroff CB, "Neurobiological effects of childhood abuse: implications for the pathophysiology of depression and anxiety,"
Arch Women Ment Health 2003 Feb;6(1):15-22.

Perry, Bruce, "The neurodevelopmental impact of violence in childhood,"The ChildTrauma Academy, www.childtrauma.org.

Perry, BD, "The neurodevelopmental impact of violence in childhood," in Schetky D & Benedek E, eds., Textbook of Child and Adolescent Forensic Psychiatry,
American Psychiatric Press, Inc., Washington, DC:2001.

Perry BD, "Incubated in Terror: Neurodevelopmental Factors in the 'Cycle of Violence,' in: Children, Youth, and Violence: The Search For Solutions, J. Osofsky, Ed.,
The Guilford Press, New York NY:124-48.

Pirraglia, PA, et al, "Trends in prescribing of selective serotonin reuptake inhibitors and other newer antidepressant agents in adult primary care,"
Primary Care Companion, J Clin Psych 2003;5:153-7.

Reuss, Alejandro, "Cause of Death: Inequality,"
Dollars and Sense, May/June 2001.

Rosmond R, "Stress induced disturbances of the HPA axis: a pathway to type 2 diabetes?"
Med Sci Monit 2003 Feb;9(2):RA35-9.

Safren SA, et al, "History of childhood abuse in panic disorder, social phobia, and generalized anxiety disorder,"
J Nerv Ment Dis 2002 Jul;190(7):453-6.

Sapolsky RM, Alberts SC, Altmann J, "Hypercortisolism associated with social subordinance or social isolation among wild baboons,"
Arch Gen Psychiatry 1997 Dec;54(112):1137-43.

Sapolsky RM, Why Zebras Don't Get Ulcers, Freeman and Company, New York, NY:1994.

Schore, Allan, "The effects of a secure attachment relationship on right brain development, affect regulation, and infant mental health,"
Infant Mental Health Journal 22;7-66:2001. Reprinted at www.trauma-pages.com.

Steptoe A, et al, "Socioeconomic status and stress-related biological responses over the working day,"
Psychosom Med 2003 May-Jun;65(3):461-70.

Masch, Maggie, "The Persistence of L.A.'s Grocery Gap: The Need for a New Food Policy and Approach to Market Development," full report at www.uepi.oxy.edu

Van der Kolk, Bessel, Alexander C. McFarlane, and Lars Weisaeth, eds., Traumatic Stress: The Effects of Overwhelming Experience on Mind, Body, and Society, Guilford Press, New York, NY:1996.

Williams DR, Fenton BT, "The mental health of African Americans: findings, questions, and directions,"
Handbook of Black American Health: The Mosaic of Conditions, Issues, Policies, and Prospects, Greenwood Press,
Westport CT: 1994.

Williams DR, Takeuchi D, Adair R, "Socioeconomic status and psychiatric disorder among blacks and whites,"
Social Forces, 71:179-94.

Ro, Ronin, Gangsta: Merchandising the Rhymes of Violence,
St. Martin's Press,
New York NY:1996.

Zinn, Howard, A People's History of the United States:
1492-present, HarperCollins Perennial Classics,
New York NY:1999.